Clinician's Guide to

Substance Abuse

Notice

Medicine is an ever-changing science. As new research and clinical experience broaden our knowledge, changes in treatment and drug therapy are required. The authors and the publisher of this work have checked with sources believed to be reliable in their efforts to provide information that is complete and generally in accord with the standards accepted at the time of publication. However, in view of the possibility of human error or changes in medical sciences, neither the authors nor the publisher nor any other party who has been involved in the preparation or publication of this work warrants that the information contained herein is in every respect accurate or complete, and they disclaim all responsibility for any errors or omissions or for the results obtained from use of the information contained in this work. Readers are encouraged to confirm the information contained herein with other sources. For example and in particular, readers are advised to check the product information sheet included in the package of each drug they plan to administer to be certain that the information contained in this work is accurate and that changes have not been made in the recommended dose or in the contraindications for administration. This recommendation is of particular importance in connection with new or infrequently used drugs.

Clinician's Guide to
Substance Abuse

David E. Smith, M.D.

President and Medical Director, Haight Ashbury Free Clinics

Medical Director, State of California Alcohol and Drug Programs

Medical Director, California Collaborative Center for Substance Abuse
Policy Research

Editor-in-Chief, *AlcoholMD.com*

San Francisco, California

Richard B. Seymour, M.A.

Director, Haight Ashbury Publications

Manager, Haight Ashbury Free Clinics Information and Training

Coordinator, California Collaborative Center for Substance Abuse
Policy Research

Managing Editor, *Journal of Psychoactive Drugs*
and *International Addictions Infoline*

Executive Editor, *AlcoholMD.com*

San Francisco, California

McGraw-Hill
Medical Publishing Division

New York   Chicago   San Francisco   Lisbon   London   Madrid   Mexico City
Milan   New Delhi   San Juan   Seoul   Singapore   Sydney   Toronto

McGraw-Hill
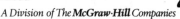

A Division of The **McGraw·Hill** *Companies*

Clinician's Guide to Substance Abuse
Copyright © 2001 by The **McGraw-Hill** Companies, Inc. All rights reserved. Printed in the United States of America. Except as permitted under the United States Copyright Act of 1976, no part of this publication may be reproduced or distributed in any form or by any means, or stored in a data base or retrieval system, without the prior written permission of the publisher.

1 2 3 4 5 6 7 8 9 0 DOC DOC 0 9 8 7 6 5 4 3 2 1

ISBN 0-07-134713-5

This book was set in Korinna by Keyword Publishing Services.
The editor was Martin Wonsiewicz.
The production supervisor was Catherine Saggese.
Project management was provided by Keyword Publishing Services.
The cover design was by Aimee Nordin.
R.R. Donnelley & Sons was the printer and binder.

This book is printed on acid-free paper.

Library of Congress Cataloging-in-Publication Data
Smith, David E.
    Clinician's guide to substance abuse / authors, David E. Smith, Richard B. Seymour.
        p. ; cm.
    Includes bibliographical references and index.
    ISBN 0-07-134713-5
      1. Substance abuse.   2. Drug abuse.   3. Substance abuse—Patients—Rehabilitation.   I.
    Seymour, Richard, 1937–   II. Title
      [DNLM: 1. Substance-Related Disorders—diagnosis.   2. Substance-Related
    Disorders—rehabilitation.   WM270   S645c   2001]
    RC564.S565   2001
    616.86—dc21   00-050080

Contents

Preface

At the beginning of a new century and a new millennium, treatment of alcohol and other drug abuse and addiction faces both crises and great opportunities. In the decades since the Second World War, America and the world have gone from being cultures with drug-using subpopulations to cultures that use and abuse drugs. Until recently, the national response to an unprecedented spread of addiction and abuse has been a draconian "war on drugs." This so-called war, supported by data-proof national and international policies, has served to criminalize and drive underground the victims of a disease.

The director of the National Institute on Drug Abuse has declared drug addiction to be a "brain disease." That declaration is supported by scientific research that consistently shows addiction to be a product of hereditary and environmental factors not unlike those found with the disease of diabetes. Yet the sufferers from the latter disease are treated while many victims of the former have found themselves in prison for the crime of being sick.

In the text of this book, the authors emphasize that there is a clear distinction between substance abuse and substance dependence, although with the progression of the disease of addiction this line is often blurred. There is also substantial debate in the field relative to these definitions, reflecting the bias and experience of proponents of different theories. As emphasized in the text, the authors believe that the evidence is clear that some substance abusers may be able to return to controlled use of their psychoactive drug, although substantial public health risks may remain. Once the individual crosses the line into substance dependence or addiction, the individual can *not* return to controlled use. Recovery from addiction can best be achieved through a substance-free lifestyle, with recovery being defined as learning to live a comfortable and responsible life without the use of psychoactive drugs.

Today populations are waking up to the fact that policies that criminalize and incarcerate alcohol and other drug users just do not make sense, either from a scientific or an economic standpoint. Economically, studies have shown that every dollar spent in treatment saves at least seven dollars in costs to society down the road. Scientifically, current advances in research on brain chemistry and epidemiological studies of addicts and abusers have clearly shown links between brain cell abnormalities and vulnerability to addiction. Further, treatment outcome results have shown that the disease of addiction is treatable, that it can be brought into remission, and that its victims can come to lead normal lives as productive members of society.

In California and other states, ballot initiatives are calling for public health rather than criminal justice solutions to the problem of addiction. Far from legalization of dangerous drugs, the call is for "medicalization" of the drug field, that is, remanding those who currently go to jail for possession or use of drugs into treatment and bringing the weight of what works to the treatment of abuse and addiction. The move toward medicalization, however, greatly increases the need for treatment availability in a field that is already overextended. Treatment centers throughout the United States are having to turn away patients in need of addiction treatment, and many have up to 50% waiting lists at a time when even more patients in need are starting to be diverted to treatment by the drug courts and other avenues of medical jurisprudence.

It is the authors' contention that the needed expansion of treatment availability can best be accomplished by educating the existing health professional community on the understanding, diagnosis, assessment, and treatment of alcohol and other drug abuse and addiction. That is why we are writing this book primarily for the physicians and other health professionals who are not addiction medicine specialists.

Within treatment circles, there is growing support for "office-based addiction treatment." This means using existing medical facilities to expand treatment availability and reduce the growing pressure on addiction specialists and specializing facilities. In a number of states and at the national level, legislation is in development and process to facilitate this expansion. With this book, the authors hope to provide a durable guide to the principles of addiction medicine that have been developed by the American Society of Addiction Medicine—one that will help nonspecialists break through resistance and stereotyping by demystifying addiction and clarifying what nonspecialist health professionals can do.

Addiction is the world's most democratic disease; it can affect anyone. Data shows that 100% of addicts do have contact with health professionals during their drug-using career. With the help of this book, nonspecialists can learn to identify addicts and potential addicts within their practice. It can help these professionals to understand the principles of diagnosis and assessment; the nature of the disease and the drugs, including alcohol and tobacco, that can trigger it; potential medical complications and sequelae; issues involving special populations such as adolescents, women, and older patients; in fine, the basics of understanding and treating the disease of addiction. It can also provide information on referral and how to get more information when needed. One of the authors' colleagues once remarked that access to information on addiction becomes critical for the physician when an addicted patient is presenting in his or her office. It is our hope that this book will provide answers and access when they are most needed.

It is the authors' pleasure to acknowledge and thank those groups and individuals who helped make this book possible. First of all, to the editors and authors of the American Society of Addiction Medicine's *Principles of Addiction Medicine*, ASAM CEO James F. Callahan, and the many colleagues whose work has become the foundation for the field of addiction medicine and whose wisdom will now contribute to the abilities of nonspecialist health professionals. Special thanks to their associate editor Bonnie B. Wilford, a long-time friend, for all that she has done for this book. To the staff and members of the California Society of Addiction Medicine, especially to director Gail Jara, for all their help, including assimilation of new information on buprenorphine treatment. To Darryl S. Inaba and the staff of the Haight Ashbury Free Clinics for giving us shelter and for being the pioneers that they all are. To all those colleagues in government, treatment, prevention, in all phases of the struggle to control addiction. And finally, to Millicent and Sharon.

Clinician's Guide to
Substance Abuse

Introduction: What is an Addict? Breaking the Stereotypes of Addiction

From his fringe of white hair to his well-tailored suit, the man is every inch a respectable pillar of the community. He is in fact a prominent doctor, a man who has saved many lives in his career. He is speaking to a conference of health professionals who are working in the field of alcohol and other drug addiction. The doctor looks down at the thick medical file in front of him on the podium and frowns. He lifts pages from the file at random and looks up, not hiding his disgust. His intense gaze takes in the audience. Then he looks down and reads off notations from the pages in front of him.

"Admitted to hospital after falling off front porch, treated for minor lacerations and released." This pillar of the community, tall and straight in a gray pinstripe suit, shakes his head and goes on. "Admitted to hospital after running car into tree beside driveway. Treated for broken collar bone and released. Treated at home by emergency medical staff after passing out under the table at a family reunion. Wife administered Valium as a sedative. Admitted to hospital..." The list goes on, hospital admissions for minor accidents and mishaps, visits from hospital personnel. Finally, he closes the file and looks once more at his audience of fellow doctors, nurses, counselors, and other health professionals.

"Would it surprise you," he asks, "to learn that this patient is one of us? a health professional? a doctor? Well, he is. Would it shock you to learn that this file is from that doctor's own hospital, the place where he was a resident, the place where he frequently performed medical examinations and operations? Would it shock you to learn that his own colleagues witnessed many of these medical mishaps, and yet over a period of years, none of them ever suggested that he might have an alcohol or other drug problem?"

Murmurs of indignation from the audience, cut short as the physician raises his hand for silence.

"Well, it doesn't surprise me," he continued. "It saddens me that no one in that entire hospital ever stepped forward. That I know for a fact, because I am that doctor. This is my medical record. Hello, my name is ____ and I am an addict and alcoholic."

She is 16 years old, a high-school cheerleader. She is a "good" girl. Never even thought about drugs, studied and got good grades, dated but did not have a steady, almost always came home in time to meet her parents' 11 o'clock curfew. Her parents had always been very honest with her, and she knew that her father had had a drinking problem and her mother had had problems with sedatives. She knew that both of them were in recovery and went to meetings on a fairly regular basis. They told her that she might have a biological vulnerability to addiction. They told her what to watch out for.

One night she went to a party where the host's parents were out of town and everyone was drinking, many for the first time. She drank too, for the first time. Some of the kids got sick, some passed out, many acted silly and some did things they felt ashamed of later. She experienced a 3-hour blackout, had no idea how she had gotten home and was relieved to see her car parked in front of the house the next morning.

She told her parents exactly what had happened, and they explained to her that blacking out was not a normal reaction for a teen drinking for the first time. She agreed and that evening accompanied her parents to her first alcoholics anonymous meeting.

He had smoked pot at rock concerts in the 60s, but he had outgrown all that. By age 35, he was a moderately successful businessman. He drank moderately, maybe a couple of martinis at a business lunch now and then, cocktails in the evening, wine with dinner. One evening in the course of a particularly taxing work situation, a colleague introduced him to a prescription stimulant to help him through an evening session with the books. The man discovered that the drug gave him the extra energy he needed to develop a competitive edge. Soon, he was relying on stimulants, and for a while his business prospered—for a while. By the time he entered treatment, his business was heavily in debt and his personal life was in shambles.

She was a woman of privilege, gracious, poised in public, the wife of a president. She could have hidden her addiction to alcohol and psychoactive medications, but in the end she didn't. Instead she gave her name to one of the most influential and effective treatment centers for addicts, ranging from the down and out to the rich and famous, like herself.

He is 14 years old and has been smoking crack cocaine since he was 11. He lives in the projects with his grandmother. His mother is doing 10 to 30 in the state pen. His father? Who knows. His pride and joy is the Uzi machine gun with which he protects his territory against other crack dealers. He has a good clientele. Most of his customers are white boys and girls from the suburbs.

What is an addict? On the face of it, that would seem to be a simple question to answer, and yet, how many of us are free from popular stereotypes? How many of us visualize the quintessential addict as a broken-down stew-bum lying in some skid row alley or shooting up in a tenderloin hotel room, mesmerized by the flashing neon sign outside the window reflecting on yellowed and peeling wallpaper? How many of us still see Johnny Machine, the Man with the Golden Arm? Stereotypes have power over us because they are hard to lose.

In reality, addicts are all of the above and more. Far from being a bottom feeder, addiction is probably the most democratic disease we have. A disease? Yes, a disease. Brought on by a combination of genetic and environmental factors, addiction is as much a product of brain wiring as it is the influences of where one lives or grew up. Statistics have shown that a vulnerability to addiction may be inherited, but it is not specific to any one race, religion or class. It has been said that an alcoholic can be hooked just as easily on single malt whisky or vintage champagne as he or she can on dollar a bottle white port. And yet, the stereotypes have held and only recently has addiction been recognized as a disease and treated as such.

With the establishment of the American Society of Addiction Medicine (ASAM), and its acceptance within the American Medical Association (AMA), the study and treatment of substance abuse has become a medical specialty, complete with texts and certification examinations. Medical experts who have been certified in the field of addiction medicine are entitled to use the appellation, F.A.S.A.M.

The legitimizing of addiction treatment has been a tremendous leap for an area of medicine that literally was legislated out of existence in the 1920s and relegated to the criminal justice system into the 1950s. In those days, the stereotypes of alcoholism and other drug addictions were very strong. When Vincent Dole and Marie Nyswander advocated for the use of methadone to treat addicts, they were ridiculed by those who saw all addicts as criminals who belonged in prison. It was only with American servicemen returning from an excruciating war in southeast Asia dependent on heroin that Dole's and Nyswander's concept was accepted and initiated on a national basis. When David E. Smith opened the Haight Ashbury Free Clinic in 1967 and began treating drug abusers, his teachers from the University of California in San Francisco said, "You were such a promising student, where did you go wrong?"

Today, addiction is being more accepted as a disease. Fearless people like Betty Ford have come forward and given addicts a human face. Research has shown that treatment does work as both a medical and an economic response to the costly devastation of drug abuse and addiction. The CALDATA study conducted by California's drug czar Dr. Andrew Mecca showed that every dollar put into treatment efforts will save seven dollars in social, medical and criminal justice costs.

The proof is there, and yet the stereotypes persist. Legislators are still convinced that all addicts are criminals and pour three times as much support into criminal justice efforts against drug abuse as they provide for treatment and prevention. Health professionals persist in casting a blind eye on the problems of patients and colleagues who do not fit their picture of an addict.

In his introduction to ASAM's *Principles of Addiction Medicine: Second Edition* (1998) National Institute on Drug Abuse director Alan Leshner, Ph.D., states that: "The reality, based on 25 years of research, is that drug addiction is a brain disease—a disease that disrupts the mechanisms responsible for generating, modulating, and controlling our cognitive, emotional, and social behavior." He adds that although most disease victims are viewed with compassion and sympathy, victims of brain diseases are not. He points out that drug use may have been voluntary at first, just as bad diet may be initially responsible for clogged arteries, but one treats the heart disease rather than berating or penalizing its victims for the dead cows or semi-solidified fat they may have eaten to cause the problem in the first place.

As with vulnerability to serum cholesterol, vulnerability to addictive disease may vary from person to person. Some may go through a long process of excessive use before crossing the line into active addiction. Others, like the teenage cheerleader above, may show symptoms of addiction with their first use of a psychoactive drug. It is known that individuals whose parents or grandparents had alcohol or other drug problems may have a heightened vulnerability to addiction. It is suspected that individuals in high risk environments, those where drinking and other drug-related activities are commonplace, may also have a heightened vulnerability. It has been demonstrated that for those who are vulnerable, the younger the person starts drinking or using, the more rapid the process of developing active addiction will probably be.

Roughly one out of every ten people in this country had, has, or will have a problem with alcohol or other drugs. As a public health problem, addiction stands alone in this country as a treatable disease for which the availability to provide treatment for all who need it simply does not exist. Increasingly, publicly supported drug treatment facilities are experiencing up to 50% waiting lists because facilities and staff at these specialty clinics are not adequate to treat the number of individuals wanting and needing addiction treatment. The situation is particularly tragic in that the point at which addicts are ready to enter treatment represents a window of opportunity that is short-lived and may not be repeated. When access to treatment is not available, the addict may not try again and may instead fall deeper and deeper into the progressive disease of addiction in a descending spiral that all too often ends in death.

Although, through the efforts of ASAM and the many state specialties, and through inclusion of addiction training and credentialling of specialty counselors, there are now addiction specialists. However, these specialists are few and far between. On their own, they cannot provide the access to treatment needed to adequately come to grips with the disease of addiction. It is therefore important for the rest of the community of health professionals to become acquainted with the nature of addiction, its myths, its stereotypes, but most important of all, its realities and the actuality of what the non-expert in addiction medicine can do to identify the problem in patients and to provide whatever intervention, care and/or referral may be necessary. San Francisco and Baltimore in particular have initiated programs that address the need for treatment on demand with access to treatment for all who need it when they need it, and these programs depend on involving the larger medical community.

Involvement of the larger medical community of non-addiction experts requires breaking down the myths about addiction and the stereotypes of addicts that now create a barrier to that involvement. The myth that addiction is untreatable, for example, can contribute to clinicians actively avoiding any involvement with alcoholics and other addicts. The truth is that addiction is treatable. The disease may be incurable in that users who have crossed the line into addiction cannot return to non-addictive use, but the disease itself can be brought into remission through programs of detoxification coupled with psychosocial therapy, abstinence and adherence to supported recovery. The myth is that addicts are down-and-outers living in slums and inhabiting a criminal underworld. The truth is that addicts may be anywhere and anyone, in the neighborhood, down the hall, in practice with you, or even in the mirror.

This book is written for the non-expert in addiction medicine. It is meant to provide a guide to the nature of the disease and can be read straight through or used as a reference when needed. Donald

Wesson, M.D., has said that most clinicians develop a need to know about drug abuse and addiction when they have patients presenting—and then they need to know, NOW! Hopefully, *Clinician's Guide to Substance Abuse* will provide that kind of reference.

The book opens with a definition of addiction that is the emerging paradigm describing the disease as it is currently seen by many clinicians. The definition is set into a context of past paradigms of addiction and some of the misconceptions that those paradigms have engendered. The opening chapter concludes with the coming together of treatment and recovery, a coming together that is legitimizing treatment as the bridge between active addiction and active recovery.

Chapter 2 provides insights into how drugs work within the human brain to produce their desired effects and ultimately, addiction. Current developments in receptor site science and neurobiology are presented to show that psychoactive drugs act by stimulating, depressing, or masquerading as the brain's various neurotransmitters. Brain function is explored, including the role of the limbic system in reward, the function of the locus ceruleus in drug craving, and the ways in which neurotransmitter site adaptations and cascades work to exacerbate addiction itself, contributing to its nature as a progressive disease. Theories of how differences in brain chemistry contribute to vulnerability and how the disease can continue to be progressive even when it is in remission are presented and discussed.

Chapter 3 talks about the basic groups of psychoactive drugs: natural and synthetic pain management drugs, sedative hypnotics, stimulants, hallucinogens and some of the hybrid drugs. Where do such substances as phencyclidine (PCP) and steroids fit into the abuse picture? How clinicians can make treatment inferences based on symptoms that indicate the type of drug ingested.

Chapter 4 then presents the signs and symptoms of addiction, providing physical and behavioral measures that can be the basis for clinical intervention, diagnosis and referral.

Chapter 5 employs and explains the basic diagnostic texts, such as DSM IV, ICD 10 and others, and how they can be utilized in planning diagnosis-driven treatment in conjunction with ASAM's patient placement criteria. (These criteria for both adults and adolescents are included as an appendix to this book.)

Chapter 6, the long chapter, presents the nuts and bolts of addiction treatment, starting with measures for dealing with potentially fatal overdose and acute withdrawal, which can also produce seizures and can be fatal. Detoxification strategies are discussed, as are accompanying medical, psychosocial and behavioral therapies up to the initiation of abstinence and introduction into recovery. Approaches include discussion of outpatient and hospital treatment, Minnesota model, methadone and other maintenance strategies, therapeutic communities, employment of antagonist and anti-craving medications.

Chapter 7 discusses the clinician's role in introducing the patient to the recovering community. Discussion of the history and nature of Alcoholics Anonymous, Narcotics Anonymous, Cocaine, Marijuana and other 12-Step fellowships, secular recovery and other approaches to ongoing abstinence and fellowship. Addiction educators such as John Chappell, M.D., have shown that the prognosis of recovering addicts increases greatly if the primary care provider takes an active part in introducing the patient to the recovering community, but this requires a knowledge of the workings of that community and the understanding that it is not homogeneous and interchangeable. There is a real need to work with patients so that they can choose the meetings and fellowships that are best for their own recovery.

In Chapter 8 it is clear that drug abuse and addiction has many sequelae. These include the most obvious, such as vulnerability to HIV disease and hepatitis B and C, and lung cancer from smoking, but also involves a wide variety of renal, hepatic, cardiovascular, and other systemic problems resulting from specific drug toxicity or compromised immune systems. There are also potential problems from non-dissolving materials used to increase the bulk of illicit drugs. These can clog capillaries and cause a variety of problems including blindness. Then there are infections to the blood and organs, as well as needle abscesses and other skin foliate complication. One recent development was the appearance of systemic botulism contracted by homeless addicts using park pond water to dilute their injected drugs.

Sharon Wegscheider, Claudia Black and Stephanie Brown pioneered the study of family dynamics and interactions in addiction. In Chapter 9, the family in addiction is explored both from the models these women developed and from a variety of other psychosocial observations. No addict exists in a vacuum. The family is involved in a variety of ways and needs to be considered in any effective treatment regimen.

Chapter 10 looks at the specific issues faced by women in addiction treatment. The work of Marty Jessup, RN, and others who have pioneered women centered treatment is discussed. The dilemmas of addiction, pregnancy, spousal abuse are explored.

As women have unique issues in addiction, so do children and adolescents. As the age of entry into drug abuse becomes lower and lower, the clinician needs to be aware of problems in a pre-teen and teen population. In these groups, differences in environment can be particularly acute. There is a great difference in working with suburban youth with present and caring parents and young dealers living within a milieu of constant violence or threat of violence and with no parental support.

Finally, the last chapter addresses such issues as nutrition counseling and explores further how non-experts can help their patients maintain a productive abstinence and recovery.

In an appendix, the authors provide information or consultation and referral resources that can be accessed personally, by phone or internet, throughout the United States.

This book is meant to provide an overview of substance abuse and addiction rather than an exhaustive and detailed exposition of the field. For those who want to do further reading on the subjects, each chapter in the book will contain a list of references and selected readings that may provide more detailed information on the specific topics that the authors have addressed. For the most inclusive and detailed presentation of substance abuse treatment state-of-the-art, the authors recommend *Principles of Addiction Medicine, Second Edition,* published by the American Society of

Addiction Medicine, Inc., 1998. For the clinician or other health professional who is not an expert in addiction medicine, the volume before you provides the basics for understanding this most pervasive and often puzzling disease.

1
Chapter One

The Nature of Addictive Disease

What is addiction? For the purposes of this book, some boundaries must be applied to the term. In recent years the term "addiction" has been applied to a number of behaviors, often referred to as "process addictions." These behaviors include compulsive gambling, compulsive sexual activity, and various eating disorders to name only a few. In this book, the authors refer in speaking of addiction specifically to addiction involving the compulsive and out of control use of psychoactive drugs. The authors do include within the scope of their work addiction to alcohol, also known as alcoholism, and addiction to nicotine in the form of tobacco. Although these are both substances that our culture has given itself permission to use in a recreational, non-medical way, they are powerful psychoactive agents that produce both physical dependency and addiction.

Psychoactive Drugs of Abuse and Their History

Psychoactive drugs are drugs that have their principal action on the brain and central nervous system (CNS). In this sense, alcohol is seen as a psychoactive drug, and alcoholism as addiction. Overeating, gambling away one's inheritance, or compulsive bungee jumping may have some similar symptoms and share a common root in human compulsive behavior with drug abuse; they may even involve some of the same brain neurotransmitter activities, but they do not specifically involve the use of psychoactive drugs, and are therefore not the subject matter of this book.

These drugs will be discussed in detail in Chapter 3: Pharmacology of Addictive Substances. For purposes of introduction, the psychoactive drugs generally involved in the process of addiction are opioids (including heroin, morphine, opium itself, and a variety of synthetic CNS pain killers), sedative-hypnotics (including barbiturates, such benzodiazepines as librium, valium, xanex, etc., and alcohol), stimulants (including methamphetamine, amphetamine, cocaine in its various forms, and tobacco), hallucinogens (including LSD, mescaline, psilocybin), and a cluster of other drugs (including the stimulant-hallucinogens such as MDA, MDMA or ecstasy, and phencyclidine or PCP which in varying dosages can act as a depressant, a stimulant, or a hallucinogen). In clinical terms, opioid drugs are sometimes referred to as narcotics. The term narcotics can be confusing, in that as a legal term it can refer to any illicit drug, no matter what its effect. For example, the Harrison Narcotic Act involves both opioid drugs and cocaine, a stimulant.

The use of substances for the purpose of intoxication is far from new. In fact, it predates humanity and can still be found in animal behavior. Cedar waxwings and other birds are prone to the ingestion of over-ripe pyracanthus berries, after which they cavort and stagger around like a troop of soccer fans. The earliest human intoxicants were probably naturally fermented plant materials. One can imagine a cave-person sampling rotting fruit found under a tree and discovering that strange things happen in his or her perceptions. One can then imagine that cave person leading his or her fellows to the tree for the world's first cocktail party. One may assume that alcohol abuse followed that same afternoon. Addiction probably took a while.

The Paradigms of Addiction

The nature of drug addiction has been a subject of human speculation at least since the days of Elizabethan England when Shakespeare touched on it in his plays. He mentions Falstaff's addiction to "sack," the British name for fortified wine. In 1779, addiction to tobacco is mentioned in a biography by Johnson. In Roman law, addiction referred to surrender to a master, or enslavement.

Given the underlying theme of enslavement, there has been a remarkable consistency to the underlying theme of drug addiction as some form of enslavement to a substance or behavior. What has varied through the years has been the cultural understanding and response to addiction. In our own time, drug addiction has been seen as willful disobedience, outright criminal behavior, a moral failing, an untreatable and incurable alteration of the human brain, the result of underlying psychopathology, and finally a unique disease.

Outmoded paradigms rarely die a quiet death. None of these views have been totally dissipated, any more than creationism has fully quit the field to theories of evolution and natural selection. While the criminal justice system continues to view addiction as criminal behavior, the military and veterans programs are still involved in whether or not addicted veterans are engaged in "willful disobedience" or are indeed "disabled," with millions of dollars in benefits at stake. In the business world, where "moral failings" are considered to be counter-productive, and at best drug abuse and addiction are generally thought to be untreatable, dismissal is often the direct result of any suspicion, especially when supported by a spot urine screen. On the other hand, a code of silence may be maintained around a senior executive's "problem."

Outmoded paradigms can lead to substituting unreal stereotypes for a true picture of addicts and addiction, and stereotyping of addicts can pose a real danger. As we have seen in the introduction, adherence, or if you will "addiction" to stereotypes often keep health professionals from recognizing addiction in either their patients or their colleagues.

Past Medical Paradigms of Addiction

■ ADDICTION AS A MANIFESTATION OF UNDERLYING PSYCHOPATHOLOGY

Medical professional and public health understandings of the nature of addiction continue to evolve, with new paradigms not fully replacing the old. Thus, in certain circles, addiction is still considered to be the result of underlying psychopathology. Utilizing that paradigm therapists may persist in wasting years working with patients who are too drunk or loaded to respond to their treatment. Such patients may indeed be suffering from a dual diagnosis of addiction and mental problems and require treatment for both, but the key, operative concept is treatment for both diagnoses.

■ ADDICTION AS UNTREATABLE

The belief that addiction is untreatable has led in the past to programs of heroin and other drug maintenance, provided with no treatment component. Such a program has been revived in Switzerland and serves the purpose of drawing in patients who would not enroll in a methadone program and therefore providing a clinical setting for their drug use, but without accompanying treatment, such drug maintenance accomplishes little else. It is the authors' understanding that the current Swiss experiment does include access to psychosocial treatment, and may therefore provide a means of engaging addicts who would not otherwise seek treatment at an early stage in their addiction.

Drug maintenance programs, providing addicts with morphine or heroin through specialized clinics, represented the state of the treatment art through the early years of this century.

Passage of the Harrison Narcotic Act in 1914 and a series of court decisions through the 1920s successively closed down these clinics, while restrictions based on the 1914 statute increasingly curtailed the ability of physicians to prescribe narcotic drugs to addicts. From that time until the early 1960s, drug treatment— which was essentially treatment for addiction to opioid drugs, i.e., narcotics—remained in the domain of the criminal justice system. Unfortunately, such treatment consisted of incarceration in federal medical facilities, where the patient/prisoners received basic medical care while detoxifying "cold turkey." Released at the end of withdrawal, these individuals often returned immediately to use, reinforcing the view that narcotic addicts were essentially untreatable.

In the 1960s, when opioid addiction spread into the middle-class youth culture, new approaches to treatment were initiated. Under the Nixon administration's "War on Drugs," the federal government established a President's Special Action Office for Drug Abuse Prevention (SAODAP) and a National Institute on Drug Abuse (NIDA), both under the leadership of the first federal drug czar, Dr. Jerome Jaffe. A few years earlier the National Institute on Alcohol Abuse and Alcoholism (NIAAA) had been established, and it and NIDA were linked to, and became partners with the National Institute on Mental Health (NIMH).

■ ADDICTION AS PHYSICAL DEPENDENCE

At that time, the prevailing paradigm of addiction focused on the drugs' effects. Addiction was characterized by the development of tolerance to one's drug and the emergence of specific withdrawal symptoms when the drug was not available or if the user attempted to stop using. Within the disease concept of addiction, physical dependence can be seen as a factor, but it is not the whole story any more than so-called psychological dependence is. As a paradigm for addiction in and of itself, physical dependence caused problems. Classical dependence, characterized by increasing tolerance and onset of withdrawal symptoms could be seen as synonymous with addiction so long as the drugs of addiction remained limited to opioids, such as heroin and morphine, and sedative drugs, such as alcohol, barbiturates, and benzodiazepines. All of these "downer" drugs produce clear-cut increases in tolerance over time and cessation in use produces identifiable withdrawal syndromes.

In the 1960s and 1970s, however, the successive spread of stimulant abuse, including the abuse of methamphetamine and cocaine, served to change the picture of what constituted addiction. The pattern of abuse for these drugs was quite different from that for opioids and sedative drugs. Here there was no steadily rising tolerance, forcing the user to take larger and larger quantities of the drug in order to achieve their desired effects. Use tended to be more episodic, with periods of abstinence occurring between binges, or "runs."

Physical vs. Psychological Dependence: Hard Drugs vs. Soft Drugs

Health professionals who were treating stimulant, and hallucinogen abusers could see that they were dealing with "addiction" that did not fit the physical dependence pattern and came up with the term "psychological dependence" to describe what they were treating. That division gave rise to designating drugs such as heroin and morphine as "hard drugs," and drugs such as methamphetamine and cocaine as "soft drugs." Given the implication that cocaine was somehow not as serious a problem drug as heroin and other "downers" may well have given a boost to the emerging cocaine and crack cocaine epidemics of the late 1970s and 1980s. The further implication was that stimulant drugs were not addictive, and that implication flew in the face of clinical treatment experience that indicated the compulsion to abuse cocaine and other stimulant drugs was at least as strong, or reinforcing if not stronger, than the compulsion to abuse heroin.

The Search for a New Paradigm of Addiction

Paradigms change when they are no longer seen to fit the phenomena that they are meant to describe. So it was in the 1980s that physical dependence, characterized by increasing tolerance and emerging withdrawal symptoms, no longer fit the experience. The addition of psychological dependence to the mix only served to further confuse the issue.

The search for reasons for addiction had focused on the substances involved and their biochemical effects, as in the statement, "Heroin produces addiction," or the designation of certain substances as "addictive drugs." In developing a new explanation for and description of addiction, the focus now turned to the addicts behavior instead of the drug's ability to produce physical dependence. The question was posed: if these drugs are capable of producing physical dependence, then why does not everyone who uses them become addicted?

A telling case in point is that of iatrogenically initiated addiction. In pre- and post-operative hospital settings, powerful narcotic pain killers, both natural and synthetic opioids are used to control pain. Often, this use produces physical dependency and the patient has to be tapered off the pain medication. Statistically, in about 9 out of 10 cases, the patient is glad to have had the pain medication but did not enjoy the side effects. The patient remembers unpleasant feelings, and though grateful, is just as happy usually quite relieved when the run of medication is over. The tenth person responds positively to the drug, thinking "This is the answer to all my problems." and actively seeks out that or similar drugs. All 10 patients have experienced physical dependence, but only the tenth has developed addiction.

In the 1960s, Dr. Elfrin M. Jellineck developed a "disease concept of alcoholism," that was based on the behavior of alcoholics, or alcohol addicts. The core of Dr. Jellineck's concept proved to fit many of the particulars of addiction to other drugs as well, including both downer and stimulant drugs. That concept provided a basis, then for a new addiction paradigm, the disease concept of addiction.

The Disease Concept of Addiction..

In developing an understanding of the current paradigm of addictive disease, let us begin with a brief statement of the concept. The paradigm is still in its formative stage and has been stated in slightly different ways. The following is, however, a composite of the concept that most addiction treatment professionals currently employ in defining and describing addiction.

■ ADDICTIVE DISEASE DEFINED

Addiction is a disease, in and of itself that is characterized by compulsive use, loss of control over use, and continued use of one or more psychoactive drugs in spite of adverse consequences. The disease is chronic, subject to relapse into active use, and thought to be progressive and potentially fatal if not treated. The disease is also thought to be incurable, but it may be brought into a state of remission through abstinence from all psychoactive substances and a rigorous program of supported recovery.

That is a one-paragraph definition of addictive disease. As the definition is highly condensed, it would be worthwhile to examine the above statements point by point and see just what they mean in this context.

A Disease In and Of Itself

Throughout its history, addiction has been viewed as many things, most recently as a symptom of underlying psychopathology. Recent treatment and recovery experience has generally shown that, while many addicts may also have mental health problems as well as being addicted, these problems are coexisting within a dual-diagnosis, of which the authors will have much more to say later in this book, than in a cause–effect relation to one another.

Compulsive Use

Compulsive use involves engaging in an activity on a regular basis: the morning cup of coffee in order to get one's motor running; the evening cocktail. Such use, in and of itself, does not constitute addiction. Many people are subject to an array of compulsive behaviors, including compulsive use of a variety of substances, but their behavior, though repetitive and often ritualized is under control.

Loss of Control

The pivot-point into addiction is loss of control. Here, the individual's use of a drug is no longer accountable to reason and will. The person who vows to go out and have one beer at the party, instead gets drunk, experiences a black-out and cannot remember.

Continued Use In Spite of Adverse Consequences

The user has passed into addiction with loss of control and now finds it impossible to avoid continued use that may lead to disaster. Here we have the smoker who continues to smoke in spite of emphysema, lung cancer and even lung removal; the stock broker who loses everything to the use of cocaine.

Chronic and Subject to Relapse

Even with treatment, the addict may experience slips and relapses into active addiction due to the chronic nature of the disease.

Progressive

A curious quality of addiction is that it is progressive in its nature. Untreated, the addict will continue to deteriorate, becoming more and more under the spell of the disease. Even in remission, the disease will become more and more severe. Various explanation have been provided for this phenomena and it will be discussed more thoroughly in the chapters on "Addiction and the Human Brain" and "Basic Pharmacology of Addictive Substances." Essentially, addicted individuals who relapse into active addiction after periods of abstinence will find the onset of the active disease more rapid with each relapse and the state worse than they may have experienced it before.

Potentially Fatal

For individuals in the grips of addictive disease, use becomes increasingly toxic, involving physical deterioration and an increasing potential for fatal overdose. At the same time, judgment deteriorates leading the addict to engage in risky and life-threatening behaviors, such as unsafe sex, use of contaminated needles, uncritical use of contaminated drugs, and other behaviors that compromise the user's immune system and leave the user vulnerable to HIV disease, hepatitis C, medication-resistant tuberculosis and other drug-related disease entities. Ability to cope also deteriorates, leading to increasingly unhealthy life situations and further encourage the onset of drug-related illness.

Incurable

Addiction can be considered incurable because once the addict has crossed the line and lost control over use, he or she can never go back to non-addictive use. In the recovering community, it is said that a cucumber can remain a cucumber, but once it becomes a pickle, it cannot go back to being a cucumber. Any attempt at controlled use will inevitably fail, as the addict falls back into the progressive disease.

Note: It should be noted that not all abuse of alcohol and other drugs constitutes addiction. Learning to use in a controlled way may work for individuals who have fallen into a non-addict abuse pattern, but in general, anyone who has to even think in terms of controlled drinking most likely has an addiction problem. One way of confirming a diagnosis of addiction is for the individual to attempt controlled use. The addict cannot maintain a non-abuse use pattern and relapses to compulsive use.

Achieving a State of Remission

Although the disease of addiction is currently considered incurable, the good news is that it can be brought into remission. In this case, remission is a state of non-use, or sobriety wherein the addict can be drug-free. Through the exercise of a supported program of recovery, the addict can also be free of drug craving, physical dependence, denial, and other aspects of active addiction and lead a productive and enjoyable life in the process.

■ OTHER ASPECTS OF ADDICTION

Besides the basic definition cited and elucidated above, there are a number of other aspects to addictive disease that are involved in any understanding of how the disease works. Some of these have been mentioned above in "a state of remission."

Denial

One of the most unique aspects of addiction is the insistence by the addict that there is no problem. It has been said that alcoholics and other addicts are incapable of seeing their own addiction. That is why intervention and confrontation are often tools in initiating treatment. A second level of denial is recognizing that a problem exists but being convinced that nothing can be done about it.

Drug Craving

Drug craving is characterized by an intense desire to resume or continue using one's drug of choice. Craving can be psychological in nature, such as a response to using cues: for example, seeing white powder or finding oneself in a neighborhood where one purchased drugs. It can also be a biochemical component of physical dependence. The nature of craving will be discussed more fully in the next chapter of this book.

Physical Dependence

The addiction paradigm that preceded the current disease model was primarily based on physical dependence, characterized primarily by the development of drug tolerance and the emergence of withdrawal symptoms any time the drug is not available.

Tolerance

Tolerance is essentially the need for more of a drug over time to achieve the same desired effects. Tolerance usually builds with the chronic use of opioid and sedative drugs as a result of biochemical adjustments to the chronic presence of these drugs in the system.

Withdrawal Symptoms

It is now clear that cessation of regular use of any psychoactive drug by a user who has developed any degree of physical dependency will produce withdrawal symptoms. These may be most physically pronounced in opioid and sedative drug including alcohol users, but variations occur with all drug withdrawal.

There are many other aspects to addiction, and these will emerge throughout the book. The above, however, constitute the most general aspects to be considered at this time.

■ THE TRIPLE NATURE OF ADDICTION

It has been said that addictive disease functions at three levels, or in three different realms: these are the physical, the mental, and the spiritual. A long-term counselor and drug abuse program director, Chuck Brissett, graphically refers to the disease as a "three-headed dragon."

In an introduction to the American Society of Addiction Medicine's manual, *Principles of Addiction Medicine, Second Edition* (1998), Alan Leshner, the current director of the National Institute on Drug Abuse, states that "Drug Addiction is a Brain Disease." Leshner's statement is true as far as it goes, however, it doesn't go far enough. Any understanding of addiction has to look beyond the biochemical. In a very real sense, addiction is like the sci-fi parasitic monsters who are capable of totally replicating their human hosts. It is the authors' opinion that any approach to addiction treatment that does not take in the spiritual and psychological aspects of the disease is doomed to failure. It is therefore incumbent upon any health professional who is treating individuals with addiction problems to look beyond the mechanics of the brain to the mind and spirit of the patient as well. This can be done by developing an understanding of the disease and of the nature and dynamics of recovery.

The Etiology of Recent Approaches to Addiction Treatment

In the physical dependence phase of addiction understanding, treatment for addiction followed two primary courses; maintenance and detoxification.

■ METHADONE MAINTENANCE

Maintenance was essentially limited to opioid addicts and based on the concept that many individuals had undergone changes in their brain chemistry as a result of their long use of heroin and other narcotics and were incapable of staying off these drugs. While not all that dissimilar to the drug maintenance practiced in this country prior to the Harrison Narcotic Act, the maintenance system developed in the 1960s was based on substituting the addicts drug of choice for a synthetic opioid.

Methadone had been developed in Nazi Germany during World War II when Hitler's supplies of opium from the Near East were cut off and there was great need for a substitute battlefield pain control drug. In the 1950s, as post-war supplies of illicit narcotics were once again becoming widely available in the United States and heroin addiction was spreading through the nations slums, two doctors, Vincent Dole and Marie Nyswander proposed that the synthetic opioid be made available to heroin and morphine addicts in order to break them free from the criminally controlled world of illicit drugs.

Like other natural and synthetic opioids, methadone would prevent the onset of withdrawal in opioid addicts. Methadone had several advantages over the use of heroin or morphine maintenance: (1) It is effective when taken orally and does not have to be injected for maximum effect. (2) It is long-lasting, requiring only one application per day to maintain round-the-clock serum levels and stave off opioid withdrawal symptoms. (3) It is difficult to synthesize and therefore its availability and use can be regulated and controlled.

On the down side: (1) methadone maintenance can be seen as merely trading one addictive opioid for another one. (2) As a longer-acting drug, methadone takes longer to withdraw compared to other opioids, making eventual detoxification from methadone more difficult than it would have been for heroin or morphine.

■ DRUG DETOXIFICATION

In an arena that saw physical dependency as the defining characteristic of addiction, the logical alternative to maintenance was removing the toxic substance or substances from the addict's body, i.e., detoxification.

In practice, the most primitive form of detoxification was merely to deprive the addict of access to drugs and allow the withdrawal process to run its course. The process came to be nicknamed "cold turkey" because one of the visible signs of withdrawal was extreme piloerection, or goose bumps, that made the withdrawing addict look rather like a plucked and not very thanksgiving turkey.

With the elimination of drug maintenance clinics in the United States, treatment of opioid addicts could only take place in prison facilities. Addicts who wanted to quit generally turned themselves in to the authorities and were "treated" in specific criminal justice facilities with a variation of "cold turkey." Such treatment centered around keeping the prisoner locked up in a locked prison hospital ward where his or her basic needs were taken care of but little effort was made to supplement withdrawal with any sort of psychosocial support. When the "clean" addicts were released following their "cure," most returned rapidly to active opioid use and dependency. This seemingly inevitable recidivism strengthened the impression that addiction is untreatable. The impression of untreatability was further augmented by depictions of addicts and addiction, such as the 1955 Otto Preminger movie *The Man with the Golden Arm,* in which Frank Sinatra gave an electrifying performance as an archetypal hopeless heroin addict.

In the late 1960s, when abuse of heroin and other opioids spread to middle-class youth, private treatment centers, mostly within the growing "free clinics" community treatment model initiated by the

Haight Ashbury Free Medical Clinic in San Francisco, were legislated into legitimacy and funded by NIMH and the newly formed
National Institute on Drug Abuse (NIDA). Most of these operated on
an outpatient basis, and many provided "symptomatic" medication for ameliorating the worst aspects of withdrawal. Aside from
these non-narcotic medications, treatment consisted primarily of
counseling sessions with "peer counselors," i.e., individuals who
had themselves been active addicts but were now clean of drugs.
Often these peer counselors were recruited from the ranks of clinic
patients and were looked upon as examples of what could be accomplished through treatment. The one problem was that such clinics
experienced high relapse rates within their peer counseling staffs.
Clinics like the Haight Ashbury Free Clinics have evolved to integrating pharmacotherapy with recovery, integrating drug detoxification with psychosocial modalities including counseling and
participation in 12-Step recovery groups.

■ THERAPEUTIC COMMUNITIES

An alternative to outpatient and drop-in clinic approach to addiction was the development of drug-free social model therapeutic
communities. One of the first of these was Synanon, founded by a
non-active heroin addict named Chuck Dederich. Synanon,
Daytop Village in New York, and other pioneer communities gave
rise to an international development of communities devoted to
drug-free and sober living. Most of these rely on the community
members to provide a living environment that is conducive to staying off alcohol and other drugs. The group process emphasizes
confrontation and works best with addicts who have a history of
criminal behavior.

Addiction and Recovery

■ THE SHORTFALLS OF ADDICTION TREATMENT

While methadone maintenance may count anyone who remains on
methadone as a treatment success, that treatment only extends to

opioid addiction, in that methadone works by both warding off withdrawal symptoms and blocking the addict's brain receptor sites to other opioids. The methadone maintenance patient is therefore still vulnerable to the abuse of alcohol and other sedative-hypnotic substances and to cocaine, methamphetamine, and other stimulant drugs.

Therapeutic communities address a wider range of drug problems, but can only influence addicts while they remain within the community.

Medical and social model treatment programs, whether they are hospital-based or outpatient drop-in, have refined their programs greatly, adding anti-craving counseling and medication, and varieties of highly sophisticated psychosocial treatment both during and after detoxification.

■ TREATMENT: THE BRIDGE BETWEEN ACTIVE ADDICTION AND ACTIVE RECOVERY

All of these approaches, however, are confounded by the chronic nature of the disease itself—addiction: cunning, baffling, powerful. The ingredient that has legitimized addiction treatment came not from the neurobiology laboratory, although great strides are being made in understanding the nature of drugs and the human brain there, but from the agony of two alcoholics who came together in Akron, OH, in 1935 and started a movement that has spawned a world-wide community of recovering alcoholics and other addicts. Much more will be said about the birth and development of this movement in Chapter 7. Suffice to say for now that in the authors' opinion the recovery movement and its clinical reflection in the Minnesota model, in coming together with addiction treatment, has legitimized addiction treatment as the bridge between active addiction and active abstinence and recovery.

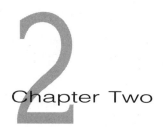

Chapter Two

History and Basic Pharmacology of Addictive Substances

Introduction: Categories of Abused Drugs

With a few notable exceptions, the bulk of psychoactive drugs that are abused by human beings fall into four general categories. These categories are: (1) opioid/analgesic drugs; (2) sedative/hypnotic drugs; (3) stimulant drugs; and (4) hallucinogenic drugs. There are abuse drugs that either fall outside these basic categories or are considered to have attributes of more than one category, and these will be discussed at the end of this chapter as specific deviations from the basic drug groupings. While the effects of psychoactive drugs may vary, they do have several things in common:

- their principal action is in the brain and central nervous system, and are therefore also referred to in the literature as "CNS drugs";
- they are able to cross the blood-brain barrier, that usually protects the brain from foreign substances, because they resemble chemicals that are indigenous to the brain;
- they all act by stimulating, depressing or imitating neuro-transmitters that are native to the human brain;
- they all produce some form of disinhibition euphoria while they are active in the brain. It is this disinhibition euphoria that tends to be the most alluring general quality of psychoactive drugs.

A Brief History of Psychoactive Drugs.............................

■ NATURAL AND SYNTHETIC DRUGS

Alcohol: The First Drug

In Chapter 1, the authors briefly mentioned a hypothetical encounter between early humanity and naturally occurring alcohol in the form of fermented fruit. Until comparatively recent times, the psychoactive drugs available for human use were all naturally occurring substances.

Fermentation

Alcohol is produced in nature through a process of fermentation, in which yeasts, a form of fungi, gather on fruit, grains and other decomposing organic materials. These yeasts feed on the sugars found in these materials and convert them to carbon dioxide gas and alcohol. In time, people learned to control the process of fermentation to produce wine, beer, mead, and other alcoholic beverages. While it may be that the initial intent was that of preserving the juices of grapes and other fruits, it is most likely that the intoxicating effects of alcohol represented an important motivation for the development of controlled fermentation. According to some anthropologists, the desire for ready intoxication via beer and other comestibles may have been a leading reason for the development of agriculture.

By the time that humanity began to shift from hunter/gatherer cultures to farming/trading cultures, the production of fermented products was already becoming a highly sophisticated endeavor. In the Paleolithic world of the Mediterranean basin, wine became a major trade item, shipped in large clay "amphorae" that can still be found en mass in the holds of ancient sunken ships.

Opium, Tobacco, and Cannabis

Opium was a *prima materium* of the ancient pharmacopoeia. In essence it is a milky substance that is toxic to the opium poppy's natural predators and is produced by the plant to protect its developing seeds. While opium may have been toxic to the insects that preyed on the opium poppy, it proved to be a highly effective euphoriant and a means of pain control, in all its forms. The earliest use of opium probably consisted of merely eating the "hip," or seed pod of the opium poppy once the flower had blown and the seeds developed. Early medical texts describe the drying and grinding of the seed pod for use in medicines. These were usually eaten, but at some point it was discovered that smoking the dried opium provided a more effective means of ingestion. For that purpose, the milky opium was harvested from the pods and cooked into a tar-like consistency that could be smoked both for medical and ceremonial/social uses.

The dried leaf of the tobacco plant was smoked in the Western Hemisphere similarly for medical and social/ceremonial use, while in the Near East, cannabis represented an early folk medicine.

Although opium and its derivatives are now classified as narcotic, tobacco a stimulant and cannabis tacitly a hallucinogen, in their original context all three had multiple medical uses within their indigenous cultures.

Coca and Khat

Leaves of the coca bush in South America and the khat bush in the Near East were chewed from time immemorial for their stimulant effects. Both plants produce powerful alkaloids that provided their users with energy and some vitamin content in locals often lacking in available foods.

Tea and Coffee

In Eastern Asia and Japan, the leaves of various plants were discovered to have stimulant properties. These were often used in infusions by monks to aid them in staying awake through long hours of meditation. It has been hypothesized that the psychoactive properties of various plants were recognized by observing the reaction of animals to these substances. A case in point is the folk-tale that coffee was discovered by the head of a Near-Eastern monastery who noticed that goats who ate a particular type of red berry were "friskier" than their fellows.

Drugs of Ceremony and Magic

Shamanism and religious practice involved the use of many early hallucinogens throughout the world. In Classical Greece, ergotomine, from which LSD-25 can be derived, was mixed with wine and herbs in a libation distributed to help celebrants see the goddess of spring as she emerged from the earth at Eleusis near present-day Athens. Shamans in South America used a number of psychoactive-containing vines and flowers to see the future and communicate with the spirit world, while their counterparts in Mexico and Central America developed rites around the peyote cactus and psilocybin mushroom.

■ THE NEXT STAGE

Cited above are only a few of the more universally used naturally occurring psychoactive substances available to a pre-industrial world. Others include the amanita muscaria mushroom, the herb wormwood, the root ginseng, to name only a few. It would seem that the world's pharmacopoeia was overflowing—and it was— with psychoactive substances, and one would think that that would have been sufficient. And so it was for a long time, in fact up into the middle ages, when alchemists developed a means for purifying active ingredients and increasing their potency.

Distillation

The basic science of distillation is relatively simple. Alchemists working in Europe and Asia in the Middle Ages discovered that when heated, the alcohol in wine, other fruit preparations, fermenting mashes of grains, and such vegetables as potatoes would vaporize and rise like spirits from their surrounding, inactive materials. In a simple apparatus, the alcohol vapor or spirits would condense on a cold surface, much like fog on a car window, and could be collected in a concentrated form.

The development of distilled spirits was probably a by-product of the alchemists incessant search for either synthetic gold or a mythical and mysterious substance they called "primum materium." In earlier times, people seem to have been content with fermented preparations containing 4–14% alcohol. Many cultures considered pure wine to be too strong to drink by itself. In Classical Greece, for example, wine was always mixed with water like a cocktail in polite society. Anyone who drank wine straight was considered something of a rounder.

The appearance of distilled spirits at anywhere from 40% to 60% alcohol was nonetheless greeted with open arms and gullets, especially in the colder regions of Northern Europe. As a result, the proliferation of distilled spirits ushered in a multi-century drunk spreading across Europe and into the Western Hemisphere with European explorers and exploiters, infecting Native-Americans who adapted the newcomers hard drinking habits.

Painters in that period recorded the grand scale of public drunkenness that was taking place around them in paintings that for a long time were thought to be allegorical depiction's of hell. Hell it probably was as populations came to grips with a spasm of drug abuse for which they were systemically unprepared. The effect of distilled spirits can be seen as a prequel to the technology-driven drug epidemics of the 19th and 20th centuries.

Extraction and Synthesis

After the development of distilled spirits, several centuries passed until the next stage. That period saw the development of new delivery systems for existing drugs, in the nature of tinctures, or substances dissolved in alcohol, such as the tincture of opium known as laudanum, and socially imbibed preparations such as absinthe, a flavored tincture of wormwood. As alchemy evolved into the science of chemistry, new ways were found to extract the active ingredients from plant psychoactives. The 19th and 20th centuries have ushered in the development of numerous purified substances: morphine and codeine from opium; cocaine from the coca leaf; and mescaline from the peyote cactus to name a few.

In 1806, Frederich Seturner isolated morphine, thus providing physicians with much greater pain control than they had with opium or laudanum. The development of the hypodermic syringe in 1853 provided a means of delivering morphine to the patients blood stream in a rapid and efficient manner. The marriage of morphine and the hypodermic came just in time for the Crimean War (1854–1856) and the American Civil War (1861–1865), providing rapid pain control for wounded combatants under battlefield conditions. An unexpected result was the creation of morphine-addicted war veterans, followed by the proliferation of morphine addiction in the general populations of Europe and the United States.

In 1874, C. R. Wright synthesized diacetyl morphine using refined morphine and acetic anhydride. The resulting product was first marketed by Bayer Pharmaceutical Products of Elberfeld, Germany, in 1898 under the trade name Heroin. Besides its use as a cough suppressant, Heroin was seen as a potential cure for morphine addiction.

Since that time, a wide variety of drugs in and beyond the four basic categories of generally abused psychoactive drugs have been synthesized, including such powerful narcotic analgesics as the fentanyls, barbiturates, benzodiazepines, amphetamines, and psychedelics. In the next section of this chapter, the authors will discuss the four categories of abusable psychoactive drugs and follow with a discussion of the drugs and other substances that fall outside these basic categories.

THE FOUR DRUG GROUPS

Narcotics/Analgesics

The narcotic/analgesic drugs have been used medically for pain relief and have been abused primarily for their ability to induce a state of euphoria and control pain. Historical accounts of opium extend to Assyrian depiction's of goddesses with poppy pods growing out of their heads from around 4,000 B.C. Opium smoking became endemic in China in the 19th century after the British began exporting the drug from large holdings in India. The Chinese "Opium Wars" were fought when the Chinese government of the time attempted to keep the drug out. China lost what the British called the "Wars of Free Trade." In Britain, opium pills of 2–3 grains were easily available from apothecaries well into the 20th century. These and the tincture of opium, laudanum, are thought to have addicted many British writers and artists of the "romantic" and "pre-Raphaelite" periods. In America, opium and cocaine were often combined in patent medicine and tonics sold by traveling "snake-oil salesmen" in rural areas. Medical educator John Morgan characterized the turn of the century opioid abuser as "A middle-aged, middle-class white woman with children."

Natural opioids, that is opioids extracted directly from opium include codeine—used for dental and other post-operative pain, laudanum, paregoric—a mild tincture of opium mixed with camphor and used primarily for control of diarrhea, and morphine. Heroin is a partial synthetic that combines morphine and diacytal acid. There are a number of synthetic opioids, including the highly powerful fentanyl (Sublimaze®), methadone—used in morphine and heroin addiction treatment, and such pain control mainstays as meperidine (Demerol®), Hydromorphone (Dilaudid®) and Oxycodone (Percodan®). See Table 2-1 for a partial listing of opioid drugs.

Medical Use of Opioids

Both natural and synthetic opioids are now, as they have been throughout medical history, the primary means of providing relief from pain and anticipatory anxiety. Along with analgesia, they induce a corresponding state of well-being or euphoria and at high doses somnolence, sometimes referred to as twilight sleep. They can also provide a sense of being immune to the effects of environmental and psychic distress, what street users refer to as "being in the wicker basket." Opioid drugs can also be effective in controlling diarrhea and coughing.

TABLE 2-1. OPIATES AND OPIOIDS

Generic Drug Name	Trade names	Schedule
Opiates (opium poppy extracts)		
Optium	Pantopon®, Laudanum®	II
Morphine	Infumorph®, Kadian®, etc.	II
Codeine (with the following)	Empirin®, Tylenol®, etc.	III
Thebaine	None	II
Semisynthetic opiates		
Diacetylmorphine	Heroin	I
Hydrocodone	Vicodin®, Hycodan®, etc.	III
Hydromorphone	Dilaudin®	II
Oxycodone	Percodan®, Tylox®	II
Synthetic opioids		
Methadone	Dolophine®	II
Propoxyphene	Darvon®, Darvocet-N®, etc.	IV
Meperidine	Demerol®, Mepergan®	II
Fentanyl	Sublimaze®	II
Pentazocine	Talwin®	IV
Levorphanol	Levo-Dromoran	II
Levo-α-acetylmethadol	LAAM®	II
Buprenorphine	Buprenex®	V
Oxymorphone	Numorphan®	II
Butorphanol	Stadol®	IV

Adapted from Inaba et al. (Ref. 1).

How They Work

The molecular structure of opioids is similar to that of certain neu-rotransmitters that occur naturally in the brain. Because of the similarities, these drugs are able to cross the blood-brain barrier and able to occupy receptor sites used by these neurotransmitters. The brain substances have been called "endorphins," which is short for endogenous morphines. The endorphins are what provide our natural pain control. They are activated when we experience pain.

If we consider pain to be a signal that something is wrong, then endorphins are the internal means of mediating that signal. The subjective sequence is more or less as follows: Say you hit your thumb with a hammer. Intense pain. The brain receives the message, "Stop hitting yourself in the thumb with that hammer!" You jump around and yell a bit. It really hurts. After a while, though, you may still feel some surface pain from damaged thumb tissue but the intense initial pain is gone. The endorphins that the pain released in the brain have attached to receptor sites that have disconnected the acute pain signal to your central nervous system (CNS), and even given a little sense of euphoria—the crisis is over.

Non-medical Use and Abuse

Opioid drugs provide a vastly amplified version of what the internal pain management messengers provide. Beyond that, the use of opioid drugs gives the addict access to the reinforcement reward system, normally reserved to reward the performance of species-specific survival behaviors. That access provides the user with an experience that the brain equates with profoundly important events like eating, drinking, and sex. As a consequence, opioid use becomes an acquired drive state that permeates all aspects of human life. This quality makes these drugs prime candidates for non-medical use and abuse. Non-medical use often involves self-medication and can be a result of medical misprescribing. Chronic pain sufferers, for example, may find ongoing relief in situations where they have been underprescribed for pain medication. The problems of chronic pain will be addressed in detail in Chapter 11.

Whether iatrogenic in nature or developed on the street within a drug sub-culture, addiction to opioid drugs can occur with any drug in this category. Street users generally gravitate toward morphine and heroin, available through illicit dealers. Middle-class addicts and health professionals find prescription opioids more available to them, but that can change over time and with changes in availability.

Ingestion of Opioids

Opioids may be taken orally in pill or liquid form, such as codeine or the many opioid-based prescription cough and diarrhea medications. They may be injected under the skin (skin popping), intramuscularly or intravenously. Injection has the added attraction of producing a "rush," i.e., a relatively immediate drug reaction that has been described by users as being like a full body orgasm.

Intravenous injection is said to produce the most intense rush. Given the expense and the frequent difficulty in obtaining opioids, and the often low potency of street drugs, economy of delivery is often a consideration. Injection provides the least waste of drug in that the substance is introduced quickly into the bloodstream without prior evaporation or metabolization taking place. With higher potency heroin, however, smoking or "chasing the dragon" is often the choice. Smoking actually is the most rapid system for delivering opioids or any other drug to the brain, even faster than intravenous injection. Further, in the light of AIDS, hepatitis C, and other illnesses that can be communicated by needle-sharing, smoking is seen by users who can afford high-quality opioids as the safest use—and often seen by them as non-addicting.

Physical Dependence

Opioid users are subject to the classic symptoms of physical dependence. These are increasing tolerance and the onset of physical withdrawal symptoms. Tolerance involves needing more of the drug as time passes to achieve the same desired results. Physical withdrawal can initiate within hours of the last use and consists of a cluster of flu-like symptoms. According to Gold, withdrawal is mediated by separate neural pathways than those involving the reward system, causing withdrawal events to be perceived as life-threatening, and subsequent physiological and psychological reactions often lead to renewed opioid use. In other words, withdrawal can be a tremendous force for continuing use, often at any cost. Many heroin smokers mistakenly believe that you can not be an addict unless you stick a needle in your arm.

Sedative-Hypnotic Drugs

Sedative-hypnotic drugs and anxiolytic drugs are CNS depressants that are used medically to reduce anxiety and/or induce sleep. They may also be utilized as anti-convulsants. Phenobarbital, for example, is often the maintenance drug of choice for seizure-prone individuals.

In general, the sedative-hypnotic family of drugs include alcohol, barbiturates, benzodiazepines and such barbiturate-like drugs as chloral hydrate, glutethimide, meprobamate, and methaqualone. New sedative-hypnotic drugs are being developed as you read, however; a list of the current drugs in these categories is to be found in Table 2-1.

■ THE DEVELOPMENT OF SEDATIVE-HYPNOTIC DRUGS

The history of sedative-hypnotic drugs has been a history of attempts to find a drug or family of drugs that produces the desired affects without the risk of dependence and debilitating or life-threatening side effects and overdoses. In the 19th century, anxiety and insomnia were treated with opiates, bromide salts, chloral hydrate (developed in 1869), paraldehyde (developed in 1882), and alcohol. Each of these substances had its problems. The bromides could cause chronic bromide poisoning, and many patients refused to take alcohol, while chloral hydrate and paraldehyde had objectionable taste and smell. As a result, the development of barbiturates was hailed as a major breakthrough.

Barbiturates

Barbiturates are all derived from barbituric acid, first obtained from uric acid and synthesized in Germany by Dr. Adolf von Baeyer in 1864. Conrad and Guthzeit synthesized the first barbiturate, 5,5-diethylbarbituric acid (barbital) in 1882. In 1903, Emile Fischer and Baron Josef von Mering introduced barbital into clinical medicine under the trade name Veronal®. Phenobarbital, which has remained the "Model T" of barbiturates, first appeared on the market in 1912 as Luminal®. Unfortunately, intoxication with barbiturates is qualitatively similar to intoxication with alcohol, and produced similar problems of abuse.

Benzodiazepines

A family of CNS depressants that has gained wide acceptance and use in the medical community is the benzodiazepines. These drugs, also called the minor tranquilizers, have been developed over the past 30 years, starting with chlordiazepoxide (Librium®), quickly followed by diazepam (Valium®). Since then, a variety of benzodiazepines have been synthesized, including alprazolam (Xanax®) and triazolam (Halcion®). The benzodiazepines may range in duration of effects and specific indications, but they are all cross tolerant and chemically similar.

Major Tranquilizers

Major tranquilizers like the phenothiazines, which include chlor-promazine (Thorazine®), are not usually subject to recreational-type abuse. Problems with these drugs most often involve mispre-scription or lack of understanding of their effects by health professionals. They are not considered to be addictive, and although a few deaths have been attributed to the ingestion of them at high doses, it is difficult to use them to commit suicide. The most notable problem with these drugs is the development of extrapyramidal symptoms, medically termed tardive dyskinesia, including facial and other abnormal movements of the head and neck, as well as such Parkinson syndrome-like symptoms as tremor at rest, rigidity, and shuffling walk.

■ ALCOHOL

Although its systemically administered medical uses have been limited to the treatment of methanol and ethylene glycol poisoning, alcohol is an excellent solvent and is used as a vehicle in many pharmaceutical formulations. It is also used topically as a disinfectant and to reduce fever through evaporation. Medieval alchemists considered it to be the "elixir of life," a title that has survived in certain European fruit brandies called collectively *eau de vie*.

While some cultures have expressly forbidden the use of alcohol, particularly some but not all Muslim cultures, most peoples have embraced this drug, giving themselves permission to use it ceremonially and recreationally, at least in moderate quantities. At the same time, alcoholism or alcohol addiction is considered to be a world-wide problem, and most cultures invoke sanctions against behavior related to alcohol over-use, such as drunk driving.

As a recreational substance, alcohol is second only to caffeine in world-wide use and second only to tobacco in health costs from abuse. In recent years, the American public has received a mixed message on alcohol's health benefits and deficits. Wine is said to help protect "moderate" drinkers from heart disease, but at the same time alcoholism is responsible for more substance-related deaths than all other psychoactive drugs combined with the exception of tobacco. While there are few pharmacotherapies for alcoholism and alcohol abuse, a manymultimillion dollar project has been funded at the University of California at San Francisco by Gallo Wine and the State of California to study alcohol neurochemistry and if possible develop effective medications based on new advances in the understanding of the effects of alcohol on brain chemistry. This important research effort is headed by Ivan Diamond, M.D., past president of the Research Society on Alcoholism. Remission from alcohol addiction was the aim of a fellowship developed in the mid-1930s, Alcoholics Anonymous, which today has a world-wide membership numbered in the millions.

Alcohol is usually imbibed in liquid form such as beer, wine, brandy, hard liquor, etc. The type of alcohol commonly consumed is known as "ethanol." It is rapidly and efficiently absorbed into the bloodstream from the stomach, small intestine, and colon. Recent studies have suggested that women have a more efficient absorption than men. In the bloodstream, alcohol is distributed to all parts of the body, including the fetus(es) of pregnant women. Alcohol is metabolized in the liver and converted to acetaldehyde by the action of alcohol dehydrogenase (ADH) and other oxidizing agents at a relatively constant rate.

■ ADVERSE EFFECTS

The effects of sedative-hypnotic overdose or intoxication are similar for all drugs in this class. Ethanol acts as a classic sedative hypnotic drug, although the quality of sleep may be reduced by its ingestion. Intoxication works to decrease most mental and physical acuity, causing lapses in judgment, unsteady gait, slurred speech, slowed reactions, and mechanical difficulty. Blackouts, that is continuing to function physically while being mentally disengaged, can occur as tissue dependence develops. Blackouts can be particularly dangerous in that users may forget how many pills they have taken and dose themselves into inadvertent overdoses. The degree of disinhibition euphoria can rapidly shift to dysphoria or even rage reactions with violent acting out. In advanced stages the intoxicated individual may pass out or in extreme cases lapse into coma requiring emergency resuscitation. Acute intoxication to any sedative-hypnotic can be a life-threatening event.

■ CHRONIC ABUSE

The effects of chronic abuse can include memory impairment, and chronic cognitive and psychomotor impairment. Tolerance develops to these drugs as the liver becomes more efficient in processing these drugs, however, the potential for a fatal overdose remains the same for these drugs. That means as the sedative-hypnotic abusers needs and uses more of the drug, he or she comes closer and closer to a potential fatal overdose. Further, as a user gets older, age-dependent tolerance also occurs, in that the effect of a sedative-hypnotic on a 50-year-old can be 5–10 times stronger than the same dose on a 20-year-old.

■ CROSS-TOLERANCE AND CROSS-DEPENDENCE

Cross-tolerance means that tolerance to any sedative-hypnotic drug will extend to other drugs in the same class. Cross dependency means that use of any drug in this class, or any opioid drug will enhance the effects and abusers may turn to other drugs in either category to either supplement their drugs of choice or stand in for them if they are not readily available.

■ SYNERGY

Synergism can occur when more than one depressant drug, including alcohol, are used at the same time. In combination, that can cause a much greater reaction than the simple sum of effects.

The liver tends to be choosy about what it metabolizes first. For example, diazepam is considered a relatively safe drug from the standpoint of being difficult to overdose on. However, if alcohol and diazepam (Valium®) are taken together, the liver becomes busy metabolizing the alcohol and the diazepam passes through to the brain at full strength. The result can be blackouts—resulting in even more use if the individual is medicating and forgets having already taken his or her medication, and extreme respiratory depression. These synergistic effects result in more than 4,000 deaths a year and almost 50,000 emergency room visits for adverse multiple drug reactions.[1]

■ HOW THEY WORK

Benzodiazepines, barbiturates, and alcohol act by stereospecifically binding to recently discovered receptors in the central nervous system. The effects of central nervous system effective sedative-hypnotics have generally been linked to this complex, which also contains the receptor for gamma-aminobutyric acid (GABA), the major inhibitory neurotransmitter in the brain and the chloride ion channel, through which chloride ions pass.[2]

GABA receptors are the main site of action for benzodiazepines in a highly complex process, but one that gives rise to the possibility of developing benzodiazepine agonists, antagonists, and inverse agonists. Benzodiazepine antagonists, such as RO15-1788 or flumazenil, may provide treatment options for both overdose and chronic abuse. The whole concept of agonist/antagonist treatment is discussed in depth in Chapter 6.

Central Nervous System Stimulants

■ THE NATURE OF STIMULANT DRUGS

Beyond the obvious of being stimulants rather than depressants, CNS stimulants have some basic differences from the two preceding groups of psychoactive substances. Although CNS stimulants can produce addiction, their users do not develop a steadily increasing tolerance. Instead, as "pre-synaptic" drugs, they exhaust the brain's own supply of stimulant neurotransmitters within the sympathetic system. This results in a binge pattern of use in which the user is forced to stop intense use periodically when the drugs no longer produce their desired effects so that the brain can replenish its supply of sympathic transmitters.

The most common stimulant drugs are caffeine and nicotine, and their use is virtually world-wide. In recent years, the deleterious effects of nicotine have come under increasing scrutiny, particularly in the United States, where it has been recognized that tobacco is responsible for at least 400,000 deaths per year. At the same time that nicotine is being increasingly censured, caffeine is enjoying what seems to be an ever increasing popularity. Perhaps this is because with increasing public health attention to the dangers of both tobacco and alcohol, it is the one remaining central nervous system drug that most people feel okay about using. Coffee shops have become the social centers of our society, and the market is increasingly dominated by chains that provide a wide variety of coffee products.

■ THE CAFFEINE CONTROVERSY (OR LACK THEREOF)

In general, coffee, tea, mate, coca-cola and other sodas are so ubiquitous that people rarely think of them as drugs. Aside from individuals who are hypersensitive to caffeine, the controversy continues on whether caffeine itself is harmful or helpful to the people who use it. There is no doubt that caffeine is a CNS drug. It is well known that many individuals are physically dependent on its daily use and will exhibit withdrawal symptoms, including headache and disorientation if their use is abruptly stopped. On the other hand, aside from the spiraling cost of cappuccinos, it may be hard to specify adverse consequences to the use of caffeine.

Writers such as Andrew Weil, M.D., in his germinal book *The Natural Mind,*[3] often contend that indigenous psychoactive substances used within cultural boundaries enhance rather than endanger the lives of their users. Plant stimulants, such as khat in Africa and the Near East and coca-leaf chewing in the South American highlands, are the most often cited as providing vitamins missing in the regional meager diets and needed stimulation for the hardscrabble existence of their users.

In teaching courses on drug abuse treatment to health professionals who may have had no personal experience with drug use and have a hard time understanding the compulsion involved, Richard Seymour asks how many are habitual coffee drinkers. Most hands usually go up. He then says, "Think about how you feel if you can't get your first cup of coffee in the morning and then multiply that. That's how the compulsive stimulant drug user feels."

■ ABUSED CENTRAL NERVOUS SYSTEM STIMULANTS

In this chapter, the authors focus on the commonly abused CNS stimulants: cocaine, including both freebase and crack, the amphetamines and methamphetamine. A drug similar in structure and effect to the amphetamines, methylphenidate (Ritalin®), and phenylpropanolamine, a stimulant vasoconstrictor that shows up in many cough and cold remedies, will also be mentioned. The most insidiously dangerous stimulant, nicotine as found in tobacco, deserves a chapter all its own, but will be discussed briefly as well.

■ A BRIEF HISTORY

Cocaine

Cocaine is derived from the coca leaf, which has been chewed for its stimulant qualities by dwellers in the South American highlands since prehistoric times. When Spanish conquistadors first encountered the Inca Empire of Peru, coca leaves were a means of exchange controlled by the emperor, himself. It is something of a miracle that coca-chewing was not imported to Europe along with tobacco use at that time. Instead, cocaine was not medically extracted from the leaf until 1860. Once the strong stimulant was isolated, however, it came into multiple use throughout Euro-American culture. Cocaine formed the original basis for coca-cola and could be found by itself or in combination with opium in a variety of quasi-medical elixirs and tonics. Its use was recommended for the treatment of asthma, hay fever, fatigue, and at least a dozen other ailments. Sigmund Freud made frequent use of it, both personally and in his practice, and was involved in what may have been the first case of iatrogenic cocaine addiction. The most common use by serious abusers was by injection. Often cocaine was injected in a combination with morphine or heroin called a "speedball." By the early years of the 20th century, cocaine abuse had become serious enough in the United States for that drug to be included with heroin in the 1914 Harrison Narcotic Act.

Today, cocaine appears in several forms: coca leaf, liquid, powdered cocaine hydrochloride, purified freebase, and crack and can be chewed, insufflated or snorted into the nose, injected (with or without opioids) or smoked.

Amphetamine and Methamphetamine

Amphetamines are a 20th century development that first came into general medical use in the 1930s for a wide variety of medical conditions.[4] During World War II, amphetamines were provided to combat troops and bomber crews who had to stay awake and alert for long periods of time in large quantities. After the war, production of these drugs remained high in most of the combatant countries, and they were readily prescribed by physicians for everything from depression to pre-finals fatigue in college students. The first serious outbreaks of amphetamine abuse occurred in Japan, where stockpiles of the drug remained at the end of the war, and in Sweden. Although some abuse had existed in the United States, the first post-war outbreak of stimulant abuse took the form of high-dose intravenous methamphetamine abuse between 1968 and 1969.

Stimulant Drug Pharmacology

Unlike the opioid drugs, which work by imitating the indigenous morphines (endorphines) and attaching directly to the endorphin receptor sites, stimulant drugs produce their effects by acting as sympathomimetic agents and thereby stimulating the release of sympathic neurotransmitters in the brain. The normal function of these sympathic agents is to implement our "fight or flight" response through release of the brain's own adrenaline or norepinephrine, with associated constricting blood vessels (vasoconstriction), increasing pulse rate and heart rate, increasing temperature (hyperthermia) and in general increasing alertness and response. These reinforcing stimulants are also directly connected with the brain's reward/pleasure center, so the satisfaction from using stimulants can be intense. One professional ball player who was introduced to cocaine at the height of his career said that the feeling from the drug was the same feeling he got when an entire stadium was on its feet shouting his name.

Nicotine

Tobacco, the primary source of nicotine was used ceremonially in both pre- and post-columbian America, imported to Europe where it was both embraced and reviled as a recreational drug, condemned by the court of James I of England, and today may be responsible for over 400,000 deaths a year in the United States alone. Contrary to popular belief, while nicotine may help focus attention, it interferes with complex brain functions including access to long-term memory and the performing of multiple attention tasks.

Nicotine and the other ingredients in tobacco have been cited as causing a variety of fatal illnesses. A study by the Centers for Disease Control (CDC) in 1991[5] listed the causes of death related to smoking with annual death toll as follows: (Cardiovascular) heart disease 150,000, stroke 26,000, other 24,000; (Cancer) lung 112,000, other 31,000; (Nonmalignant Pulmonary Disease) COPD 62,000, other including pneumonia and influenza 21,000; for a total of 426,000 fatalaties a year directly attributable to tobacco. Further, CDC points out that tobacco is also responsible for an annual death rate of 53,000 per year among non-smokers affected by smoke in their immediate environment. All of the above should make it imperative for health professionals to exercise their influence in intervening on patients who are still smoking.

Pharmacologically, tolerance to tobacco develops quickly but once established levels of smoking may remain about the same throughout one's smoking career. A withdrawal syndrome has been well established. Withdrawal symptoms may vary but can include craving for nicotine, irritability, frustration, anger, anxiety, depression, difficulty concentrating, restlessness, and increased appetite. Although nicotine withdrawal is highly distressing, may continue for weeks, and compulsion to resume use may remain high for an extended period of time, and weight gain may be daunting, it is not life-threatening. Detoxification can be an extenuated process of reversing neuronal adaptation to nicotine however.

Although nicotine is also absorbed into the bloodstream through chewing and the use of snuff, inhaling cigarette smoke provides the most rapid brain access. Nicotine can also be absorbed through the skin, facilitating the use of skin patches. It is readily absorbed through the stomach, but first-pass digestion in the liver greatly decreases the amount reaching the brain from the stomach. Patients utilizing nicotine gum are therefore now advised to mixing the gum with saliva and lodging it between cheek and gum to facilitate absorption through the buccal mucosa.

Use of tobacco is bolstered by the positive reinforcement of producing euphoria and maintained by the negative of rapid onset withdrawal symptoms as soon as nicotine levels decline below the brain's accustomed levels that are quickly relieved by the ingestion of nicotine.

■ SPEED KILLS (THE EFFECTS OF AMPHETAMINE/ METHAMPHETAMINE)

Stimulants promote the release of the brain's energy chemicals. On the short term, this can result in increased wakefulness and alertness, giving the occasional or situational user a performance edge. It was that edge that led science writers in the late 1940s to laud amphetamines as a wonder drug. Unfortunately, these drugs also deplete the brain's own adrenaline or norepinephrine chemicals, induce a drug-based paranoia, and trigger intense craving for more drug. Cocaine in particular blocks the reuptake of norepinephrine by the brain cells in which they are usually stored, creating a cerebral chain reaction until the chemicals are metabolized. The net result is the same—overstimulation of the brain followed by depletion and depression.

■ PREVENTION EFFORTS

In keeping with their stimulant nature, cocaine and the stimulants produce a very rapid onset of abuse. Prevention efforts brought the term, "speed kills." Rock musician Frank Zappa filmed a TV spot wherein he said, "Kids, if you keep using speed you'll end up just like your parents."

The most effective amphetamine/methamphetamine prevention agent, however, proved to be the intravenous users themselves. These individuals tended to be walking, acting-out negative advertisements of their drug. Anorexia left them skeletal while stimulant psychosis turned them into violent victims of delusional paranoia, a danger to themselves and others.

While these efforts were effective to some extent, it became evident in the late 1960s that not only illicit manufacture of methamphetamine but the production and subsequent diversion of pharmaceutical psychoactive drugs were both out of control and the government and industry took steps to remedy the growing problem. At the end of this chapter, you will find a section on drug legislation as it has tried to cope with the changing picture of drug abuse in the United States.

Hallucinogens

While opioids and sedative-hypnotic drugs evolved primarily as medical substances for dealing with physical and psychic pain, and stimulants developed as recreational and performance-enhancing substances, hallucinogens had their role primarily within the realms of religion and magic. Throughout prehistory, history, and on into our own century, hallucinogenic substances have been utilized, often depending on the degree of sophistication of the culture in which they are being used, as a means of establishing contact with the spirit world, the realm of the gods, or the deeper reaches of the human subconscious. Shamans have employed plant and mineral hallucinogens, often within the context of highly complex ritual to establish a point of contact between their people and their people's deities, or at least the supernatural forces that may effect their individual and collective lives.

Ethnobotanists have classified hundreds of plant hallucinogens, the majority of these originating in the rain-forests of South America. In this chapter, however, the focus will be on the five categories of hallucinogens classified by Goodman and colleagues:[6]

1. LSD-like drugs, including mescaline, psyilocybin, and psilocin;
2. drugs that probably are LSD-like, such as DMA, DOM, and DMT;
3. drugs that probably are LSD-like and have other properties, such as MDMA, MDA, and other amphetamine derivatives;
4. drugs that probably are not LSD-like, such as 5-hydroxytryptophan; and
5. drugs that are not LSD-like, such as scopolamine and delta 9-THC.

A list of the drugs in these categories follows in Table 2-2.

■ **THE HISTORY AND NATURE OF HALLUCINOGENS**

The Goodman and colleagues classification obviously utilizes LSD, or lysergic acid diethylamide as the base measure of hallucinogens. This LSD-centricity most likely relates to the status of that drug as the most widely discussed and the most notorious of hallucinogens.

Although LSD or lysergic acid diethylamide was a relatively recent discovery, dating from 1943 when Dr. Albert Hofmann, a

TABLE 2-2. HALLUCINOGENIC DRUGS

LSD-like drugs
Indolealkylamines
Lyseric acid diethylamide (LSD)
Psilocybin
Psilocyn
Phenylethylamines
Mescaline
Peyote
Drugs that probably are LSD-like
Diethyltryptamine (DET)
Dimethyltryptamine (DMT)
Drugs that probably are LSD-like and have other properties
Phenylisopropylamines
3,4-Methylenedioxyamphetamine (MDA)
3,4-Methylenedioxyethamphetamine (MDEA)
5-Methoxy-3,4-methylenedioxymethamphetamine (MDMA)
3-Methoxy-4,5-methylenedioxyamphetamine (MMDA)
Drugs that probably are not LSD-like
5-Hydroxytryptophan
Drugs that are not LSD-like
Mappine
Nutmeg, mace
Morning glory seeds
Scopolamine

Adapted from Gilman et al. (Ref. 6).

chemist at Sandoz Laboratories in Bazel, Switzerland, accidentally ingested a small quantity of a substance he had first synthesized in 1938, its most active component, ergotomine, had a long history as a psychoactive agent. Occurring naturally as a rye-grain mold, ergotomine was featured in mystic potions in the classical world. In the middle ages, when its applied use had been forgotten, the hallucinogenic effects of ergotomine contamination in the bread supplies of entire communities was blamed on witchcraft and demonic possession.

Western scientific interest in hallucinogens was rekindled in the 19th century by poets and anthropologists observing and then participating in ceremonial rites involving psychoactive substances in a variety of cultures. Mescaline, the active ingredient in the peyote cactus used by religious sects in Mexico and the American Southwest, was isolated in 1856 and by the turn of the century was available for research by the likes of Sigmund Freud,

William James, and Havelock Ellis. It was, however, the discovery of what Dr. Hofmann considered the most powerful psychic drug that induced tremendous scientific and popular interest in hallucinogen research.

With the advent of LSD availability, perception of these drugs underwent a process of evolutionary models. The first of these models was the psychotomimetic. This treated the drug experience as a form of psychosis, permitting researchers to study psychotic symptoms in non-psychotic subjects. The psychotomimetic model was followed, though not necessarily superseded, by the hallucinogenic model, which treated LSD and mescaline as tools for studying the mechanisms of perception, and the therapeutic model, which involved the use of these drugs in the treatment of alcoholism, other forms of addiction and mental health problems. Finally, there came the psychedelic model, which maintained that under proper conditions the drug experience would be one of enlightening and productive consciousness expansion. It was with the psychedelic model that the use of LSD and other hallucinogens spread from the laboratory into the community.

■ ACUTE AND CHRONIC EFFECTS

The adverse effects of hallucinogens are generally divided between acute and chronic, or long-term. The acute effects, often referred to as "bad trips," occur as direct negative results of hallucinogen ingestion and involve such elements as frightening images and thoughts, fear surrounding loss of control, and fear of losing one's mind.

Acute Effects

In 1967, David E. Smith, M.D., identified the adverse effects of hallucinogens as "largely psychological in nature," and classified them as either acute toxicity, effects occurring during the use of the drug, or chronic after-effects.[7] Although there have been some occurrences of physiological consequences, particularly with MDMA, these have been primarily of an idiosyncratic nature, while in most cases the adverse effects of these drugs still appear to be psychological in their nature.

The acute toxic effects take many forms. Often individuals knowingly take a hallucinogenic drug and find themselves in a state of anxiety as the powerful hallucinogen begins to take effect. They were aware that they had taken a drug, but felt that they could not control its effects. This condition is similar to that of not being able to wake up from a threatening dream. Some users experiencing a bad trip try to physically flee the situation, giving rise to potential physical danger. Others may become paranoid and suspicious of their companions or other individuals.

Not all acute toxicity is based on anxiety or loss of control. Some people taking hallucinogens display decided changes in cognition and demonstrate poor judgment. They may decide that they can fly, and jump out of a window. Some users are reported to have walked into the sea, feeling that they were "at one of the universe." Such physical mishaps have been described within the acid culture as "being God, but tripping over the furniture." Susceptibility to bad trips is not necessarily dose related, but can depend the experience, maturity, and personality of the user as well as "set and setting," i.e., the circumstances and the environment in which the trip takes place. Sometimes the individual will complain of unpleasant symptoms while intoxicated and later speak in glowing terms of the experience. Negative psychological set and environmental setting are the most significant contributing factors to bad hallucinogenic trips.[8]

Talkdowns of most acute toxicity reactions can be accomplished without medication or hospitalization. Paraprofessionals with psychedelic drug experience have been particularly effective at such sites as large rock concerts. In the talkdown approach, one should maintain a relaxed, conversational tone aimed at putting the individual at ease. Quick movements should be avoided. One should make the patient comfortable, but not impede their freedom of movement. Let them walk around, stand, sit, or lie down. At times, such physical movement and activity may be enough to break the anxiety reaction. Gentle suggestion should be used to divert patients from any activity that seems to be adding to their agitation. Getting the individual's mind off the frightening elements of a bad trip and onto positive elements is the key to the talkdown.

An understanding of the phases generally experienced in an hallucinogenic drug trip is most helpful in treating acute reactions. After orally ingesting an average dose of 100–250 µg of LSD, the user experiences sympathomimetic, or stimulant responses, including elevated heart rate and respiration. Adverse reactions in this phase are primarily managed by reassurances that these are normal and expected effects of psychedelic drugs. This reassurance is usually sufficient to override a potentially frightening situation.

From the first to the sixth hour, visual imagery becomes vivid and may take on frightening content. The patient may have forgotten taking the drug, and given acute time distortion, may believe this effect will go on forever. Such fears can be dispelled by reminding the individual that these effects are drug induced, by suggesting alternative images and by distracting the individual from those images that are frightening.

In the later stages, philosophical insights and ideas pre-dominate. Adverse experiences here are most frequently due to recurring unpleasant thoughts or feelings that can become overwhelming in their impact. The therapist can be most effective by being supportive and by suggesting new trains of thought.

The therapist's attitude toward hallucinogens and their use is very important. Empathy and self-confidence are essential. Anxiety and fear in the therapist will be perceived in an amplified manner by the client. Physical contact with the individual is often reassuring, but can be misinterpreted. Ideally, the therapist should rely on intuition rather than pre-conceptions.

Wesson and Smith[9] noted that medication may be necessary and should be given either after the talkdown has failed or as a supplement to the talkdown process. During the first phase of intervention, oral administration of a sedative, such as 25 mg of chlordiazepoxide (Librium®) or 10 mg of diazepam (Valium®), can have an important pharmacological and reassuring effect.

During the second and third phases, a toxic psychosis or major break with reality may occur in which one can no longer communicate with the individual. If the individual begins acting in such a way as to be an immediate danger, antipsychotic drugs may be employed. Only if the individual refuses oral medication and is out of behavioral control should antipsychotics be administered by injection. The Rock Medicine Unit of the Haight Ashbury Free Clinics, which has treated well in excess of a thousand bad trips over a 23-year period, uses 2 mg of Ativan, a short-acting benzodiazepine, and 2 mg of Haldol, an antipsychotic, intramuscularly. Any medication, however, should only be given by qualified personnel. If anti-psychotic drugs are required, hospitalization is usually indicated. It has been found at the Haight Ashbury Free Clinics, however, that most bad acid trips can be handled on an outpatient basis by talkdown alone.

As soon as rapport and verbal contact are established, further medication is generally unnecessary. Occasionally, an individual fails to respond to the above regimen and must be referred to an inpatient psychiatric facility. Such a decision must be weighed carefully, however, as transfer to a hospital may of itself have an aggravating and threatening effect. Hospitalization should only be used as a last resort if everything else has failed.

■ CHRONIC HALLUCINOGENIC DRUG AFTEREFFECTS

Chronic hallucinogenic drug aftereffects present situations wherein a condition that may be attributable to the ingestion of a toxic substance occurs or continues long after the metabolization of that substance. With the use of hallucinogens, four recognized chronic reactions have been reported: (1) prolonged psychotic reactions; (2) depression sufficiently severe so as to be life-threatening; (3) flashbacks; and (4) exacerbation of pre-existing psychiatric illness. Recently, a fifth chronic reaction has been listed in the DSM-IV, post-hallucinogen perceptual disorder.

Some people who have taken many hallucinogenic drug trips, especially those who have had acute toxic reactions, show what appear to be serious long-term personality disruptions.

These prolonged psychotic reactions have similarities to schizo-phrenic reactions and appear to occur most often in people with pre-existing psychological difficulties, such as primarily pre-psy-chotic or psychotic personalities. Hallucinogenic drug-induced personality disorganization can be quite severe and prolonged. Appropriate treatment often requires anti-psychotic medication and residential care in a mental health facility followed by outpa-tient counseling.

At the Haight Ashbury Free Clinics, it has been noted that some of the clients self-medicated their hallucinogenic-precipi-tated psychotic episodes with amphetamines.[10] Often this self-medication with amphetamines resulted in the development of amphetamine abuse, followed by secondary heroin, barbiturate or alcohol abuse patterns to ameliorate the side effects of the amphe-tamines. Thus, in certain patients, chronic psychological pro-blems induced by LSD and other hallucinogenic drugs led to complicated patterns of polydrug abuse that required additional treatment approaches.[11]

■ FLASHBACKS

By far the most ubiquitous chronic reaction to hallucinogens is the flashback. Flashbacks are transient spontaneous occurrences of some aspect of the hallucinogenic drug effect occurring after a period of normalcy that follows the original intoxication. This per-iod of normalcy distinguishes flashbacks from prolonged psycho-tic reactions. Flashbacks may occur after a single ingestion of a psychedelic drug, but more commonly occur after multiple psy-chedelic drug ingestion.

Flashbacks are a symptom, not a specific disease entity. They may well have multiple causes, and many cases called flashbacks may have occurred although the individual had never ingested a psychedelic drug. Some investigators have suggested that flash-backs may be due to a residue of the drug, retained in the body and released into the brain at a later time. Although this is known to happen with phencyclidene (PCP) and drugs similar to it, there is no direct evidence of retention or prolonged storage of such psychedelics as LSD.

Individuals who have used psychedelic drugs several times a month have indicated that fleeting flashes of light and afterimage prolongation occurring in the periphery of vision commonly occur for days or weeks after ingestion. Active and chronic psychedelic drug users tend to accept these occurrences as part of the psychedelic experience, are unlikely to seek medical or psychiatric treatment and frequently view them as "free trips." It is the inexperienced user and the individual who attaches a negative interpretation to these visual phenomena who are likely to be disturbed by them and seek medical or psychiatric help. While emotional reactions to the flashback are generally contained with the period of the flashback itself, prolonged anxiety states or psychotic breaks have occurred following a frightening flashback. There is no record of flashback activity specifically attributable to hallucinogenic drug use occurring more than a year after the individual's last use of a psychedelic drug. [12,13]

■ CHRONIC CONSEQUENCES OF HALLUCINOGEN USE

The long-term study of adverse hallucinogenic drug reactions has revealed the existence of low prevalence, but quite disabling chronic consequences of LSD use. Of particular concern is the posthallucinogen perceptual disorder (PHPD). With PHPD, individuals describe a persistent perceptual disorder which they describe as being like living in a bubble under water. They also describe trails of light and images following movement of their hands, and often describe living in a purple haze. This perceptual disorder is aggravated by any psychoactive drug use, including alcohol and marijuana, and is distinguished from flashbacks, which are episodic rather than chronic phenomena. With the PHPD, the individual often experiences anxiety, even panic, and becomes phobic and depressed. With the PHPD sufferers, our experience has been that individuals do not have a disturbed psychiatric history prior to the onset of psychedelic drug use and that the PHPD can occur even after a single dose.

With the more severe, prolonged hallucinogen reactions, such as an LSD precipitated schizophrenic reaction, or severe depressive disorder, individuals almost always have a premorbid psychiatric history and require inpatient treatment. With the prolonged psychotic reactions, antipsychotic medication is required, and with the prolonged depressive reactions, antidepressant medication is required. A major concern involves teenagers with depressive reactions to psychedelic use that may result in severe depression culminating in suicide.

With the post-hallucinogen perceptual disorder, drug-free recovery with supportive counseling is often adequate treatment, although recovery may take several months and anti-anxiety medication may be needed to treat the secondary anxiety and panic disorder which develops when the individuals feel that they are irreversibly brain-damaged and will never see normally again.

■ OTHER CONCERNS

There are many variations on the above, particularly with phencyclidine, a mind–body disassociative drug that can act as a stimulant, a depressant, and a hallucinogen depending on the dosage. These will be discussed in another chapter on treatment and assessment. Suffice to say, the etiology and pharmacology of hallucinogenic drugs is varied and involves a number of differing symptoms and sequelae.

The Harrison Narcotic Act, the Controlled Substances Act, and Other Drug Legislation

The development of psychoactive drugs has been accompanied in the past two centuries by corresponding development of legislation in the United States and to some extent in other countries designed to somehow control the abuse of such drugs. The earliest law appears to have been a statute forbidding the use of opium by Chinese, enacted in San Francisco in 1875. In his excellent history, *The American Disease: Origins of Narcotic Control,*[14] David F. Musto, M.D., traces the development of legislation and statute to the development of the Harrison Narcotics Act of 1914, initiated as a response to international opium controls and to a growing epidemic of cocaine addiction, as the first national drug control measure. There followed several decades of court cases culminating in the virtual banning of heroin and tight control of cocaine in the United States. Drug legislation at the mid-century mostly involved the banning of drugs as their abuse became recognized as problematic, such as marijuana in 1937 and LSD in 1966.

During the war years, realistically extending from 1937 into the early 1950s, most of the overseas routes for illicit drugs were effectively cut off. Major interdiction efforts were maintained by the federal government and a variety of international bodies. At home a national prevention program painting dire consequences from any drug use helped to keep consumption within a few small subcultures. The picture began to change as writers, and then young people in general began experimenting with marijuana and stimulants, and not experiencing the dire immediate consequences that had been predicted, moved on to other drugs as well.

By the end of the 1960s, production, prescribing and diversion into illicit markets of not only amphetamines but pharmaceutical psychoactive drugs in general had gotten totally out of hand. In a cooperative effort, the medical community, the law enforcement community and drug manufacturers worked together and produced the Controlled Substances Act of 1970. That act provided four primary means of regulating drug distribution:

- mechanisms for reducing the availability of controlled substances,
- procedures for bringing a substance under control,
- criteria for determining control requirements, and
- obligations incurred by international treaty arrangements.

Primarily, the act created five drug schedules on the basis of abuse potential vs medical use, with Schedule I containing heroin, all the hallucinogens then known including marijuana, and other substances with high abuse potential and no accepted medical use. The remaining schedules provide prescribing procedures and restrictions on the same basis, with cocaine, at high abuse potential but some medical use in Schedule II, requiring triplicate prescriptions and other safeguards, down to paregoric and other low abuse potential drugs requiring minimal safeguards in Schedule V. The act also contained nine major control mechanisms imposed on the manufacturing, purchasing, and distribution of substances listed by the act:

- *Registration of Handlers.* Under the act, all handlers, such as exporters, importers, manufacturers, hospitals, researchers, and physicians must be registered by the Drug Enforcement Administration (DEA). This allows the DEA to check diversion by refusing to register persons and companies that have illegally diverted drugs from legitimate stocks in the past.
- *Record Keeping Requirements.* The act sets rules for record keeping of quantity, purchases, sales, and inventories of drugs. This makes it possible to trace the path of a drug, from importation or manufacture to dispensing.
- *Quotas on Manufacturing.* The act empowers the DEA to limit the quantity of controlled substances in Schedules I and II that can be legally produced during a year.
- *Restrictions on Distribution.* The DEA is also empowered to monitor the distribution of drugs from manufacturers, importers, exporters, and dispensers to each other. Schedule I and II drugs are more tightly controlled by special monitoring.
- *Restrictions on Dispensing.* Dispensing to the user, whether a patient or a research subject, is controlled, especially with Schedule I and II drugs. Physicians must follow rules

governing the writing of prescriptions and the reordering of prescriptions.

- *Limitations on Imports and Exports.* The act contains strict limitations on international transactions involving drugs in Schedule I or II, with most deals requiring DEA approval. Similar transactions involving other drugs must be made with prior notice but not approval from the DEA.
- *Conditions for Storage of Drugs.* The act empowers the DEA to demand certain security requirements be met for premises which contain controlled substances, including construction details like reinforced concrete walls, alarm systems, and vaults.
- *Reports of Transactions to the Government.* The act requires that periodic reports regarding transactions of certain drugs be submitted to the DEA. The monitoring of Schedule I and II drugs is carried out by the Automation of Reports and Consolidated Orders System (ARCOS) a government agency computer system.
- *Criminal, Civil, and Administrative Penalties for Illegal Acts.* The act sets criminal penalties for drug trafficking, which are different from penalties for possession of drugs for personal use. Not all of these controls are applicable to drugs listed in every Schedule. Whether they apply or not depends on the drug and its schedule classification.

Scheduling a drug, however, is a complicated and lengthy ordeal, taking months or even years to accomplish, as was the case with MDMA, which has been on emergency Schedule I status since 1984. In 1985, the Drug Enforcement Agency (DEA) was provided with an emergency scheduling authority, meaning that a drug could be scheduled prior to formal scientific analysis if the drug had a strong potential for abuse. The Anti-Drug Abuse Act of 1986 included information that dealt specifically with the problem of clandestinely manufactured analogs of controlled Substances. The Controlled Substance Analogue

Enforcement Act of 1986 states that analogs of controlled substances are to be considered exactly like the controlled substance itself. That is to say, a drug that has a molecular structure similar to a controlled substance is itself a controlled substance. Further refining of the national drug laws continue to this day, and have a definite influence on addiction treatment, as we will see in subsequent chapters of this book.

REFERENCES

1. Inaba DS, Cohen WE, Holstein ME: *Uppers, Downers, All-Arounders,* 3d ed. Ashland, OR: CNS Publications, Inc., 1997.
2. Juergens SM, Cowley D: The pharmacology of sedative-hypnotics, in: Graham AW, Schultz TK, Wilford BB (eds.), *Principles of Addiction Medicine,* 2nd ed. Chevy Chase, MD: American Society of Addiction Medicine, 1998, p. 117.
3. Weil A: *The Natural Mind.* Boston: Houghton Mifflin, 1972.
4. Craig RJ, Weddington WJ: Stimulants and cocaine, in: Miller NS (ed.), *Principles of Addiction Medicine.* Chevy Chase, MD: American Society of Addiction Medicine, 1994.
5. Centers for Disease Control: Smoking-attributable mortality and years of potential life lost—United States. *Morbidity and Mortality Weekly Report* 40: 1991; 62–71.
6. Gilman AG, Goodman LS, Rall TW, et al.: *Goodman & Gilman's The Pharmacological Basis of Therapeutics,* 8th ed. New York: Macmillan, 1990.
7. Smith DE: Editor's Note. *Journal of Psychoactive Drugs,* 1967; 1(1): 1–5.
8. Smith DE, Seymour RB: Dream becomes nightmare: adverse reactions to LSD. *Journal of Psychoactive Drugs,* 1985; 17(4): 297–303.
9. Wesson DR, Smith DE: Psychedelics, in: Schecter A (ed.), *Treatment Aspects of Drug Dependence.* West Palm Beach, FL: CRC Press, 1978.
10. Seymour RB, Smith DE: *MDMA.* San Francisco: Partisan Press, 1986.

11. Smith DE, Wesson DR: Editor's Note. *Journal of Psychoactive Drugs*, 1975; 7(2): 111–114.
12. Seymour RB, Smith DE: *The Physician's Guide to Psychoactive Drugs*. New York, London: The Haworth Press, 1987.
13. Seymour RB, Smith DE, Inaba D, et al.: *The New Drugs: Look Alikes, Drugs of Deception and Designer Drugs*. Center City, MN: Hazelden, 1989.
14. Musto, DF: *The American Disease, Origins of Narcotic Control*, Expanded ed. New York: Oxford University Press, 1987.

3

Chapter Three

Addiction and the Human Brain

Introduction: The Neurochemistry of Addiction

The human mind is an amazing piece of work that can only be approached in a sense of awe and wonder. Today, we may believe that the mind is a function of the brain, but it may be equally true that the brain is an instrument of a mind that is more than the sum of its flesh and blood parts. As far as we know, the mind is the only thing that can conceive of and encompass both eternity and infinity. Einstein set the speed of light as the quintessential velocity, but thought can travel to the farthest known galaxy in an instant. In essence, for all we know, the mind remains a great mystery.

Neurochemistry is only the most recent language for describing how the brain functions, and it is the means by which we try to understand the workings of drugs in the brain. Drugs may have a profound effect on the brain's function, but it is a crude effect. Think of the brain as a well-tuned piano played by the mind. Mind, in its white tie and tails sits down at that piano brain and plays a Rachmaninoff piano concerto: subtle blendings of keys and resonances. Then, a stumbling clown lurches onto the stage and sits down. He is wearing boxing gloves and pounds the keys. In both cases there is sound.

Psychoactive drugs act on the brain in three ways: they stimulate the release of certain neurotransmitters, they inhibit the release of certain neurotransmitters, or they bind with the receptor sites designed for certain other neurotransmitters. These drugs are abused specifically for their actions on the brain's receptors and neurotransmitters.[1]

Through science, the treatment field has learned much more about the nature of addiction. It is now known, for example, that addiction is a mid-brain phenomenon. Both denial and recovery are learned activities that involve the cerebral cortex, but addiction itself is within the province of the primitive brain.

Through Alcoholics Anonymous and the recovering community, the treatment field is learning that long-term abstinence and recovery are possible if the addict's craving can be kept at bay long enough for that individual to overcome denial and learn the process of recovery.

Regarding the roles of environment, genetics and predisposition in the development of addiction, it is our view that addiction equals genetics plus environment. Over time, anyone given high enough doses of a drug may become addicted to it. When a person has a genetic predisposition, or when use starts in early adolescence addiction happens sooner and with greater ease.

The importance of a family history of alcoholism and addiction in predicting vulnerability to addictive disease continues to be significant, while the spread of drug availability and use over the past few decades bears witness to the important role of environment. Today, there are an estimated 30 to 40 million chemically dependent individuals in the United States. In 1962, approximately four million people had been exposed to illicit drugs. By 1992, that figure had risen to 80 million.[2] There has also been a major increase in Axis I psychiatric disorder among young people.

In his *Divine Comedy,* Dante refers to the inhabitants of the lowest levels of hell as *those who yearn for what they most fear.* That is a good description of people suffering from addictive disease. Addiction is a disease that is characterized by compulsion, loss of control, and continued use in spite of adverse consequences. The disease is progressive and can be fatal if not treated, and it is fueled by craving "for what they most fear." In the 12-step world, it is said that one drink is too many, while a million are not enough. Alcoholics do not react to alcohol the way that non-alcoholics do. This is because, for the alcoholic, the first drink acts as a trigger, converting craving into an overwhelming need for alcohol. The mechanisms of craving are not clearly understood, but the dynamic seems to hold true for those addicted to cocaine, heroin, tobacco, and other drugs as well as for alcohol.

The Human Brain

Anything that is said about the brain and its functioning is at best a metaphoric paradigm that changes with each new research revelation. More has probably been learned about how the brain functions in the last 20 years than was known in all of previous history, and what is now known is changing at an accelerating rate. In that dynamic electro-chemical system, brain physiology involves a variety of cells that communicate with one another via neurotransmitters.

■ BRAIN CELL COMMUNICATION

Brain cells, or neurons are composed of a nucleus located within the main body of the cell, axons which extend from the body as branches of the cell, and dendrites. Brain cells do not touch one another. Instead, the cell's axons are juxtaposed to neurotransmitter receptor sites on the dendrites of adjoining cells. The axons can be extremely long. Some extend up to 4 ft, all the way from the brain to the base of the human spinal column. At the end of each axon, as many as 10,000 or more branches, each of which can make contact with a different receiving neuron, providing a great diversity of possible neuron interconnections. Correspondingly, up to 10,000 or more dendrites on each neuron can receive electrochemical input from many neurons. According to Solomon Snyder, all thinking and feeling is a consequence of the 10 billion or more neurons in the brain talking to each other.[3]

■ A MODEL OF BRAIN DYNAMICS

In a model of what takes place, an impulse arises in the dendrite or cell body and then travels down the length of the axon by an electrochemical process. According to Snyder, "The interior of a resting neuron is electrically negative with respect to its exterior, but when a neuron is excited, the electrical potential across the cell membrane is abolished, and the cell's interior may even develop a weak positive charge." A complex series of actions, involving the concentration of sodium ions in the cell and initiating a wave of electronic activity traveling the length of the cell, results in the release of neurotransmitters that are stored within the cell. These electrochemical messengers cross the synaptic cleft, or the space between the axon and the adjoining dendrite's receptor sites. That connection is called a synapse. In the course of normal brain communication, once the neurotransmitters have interacted with the receptor sites on adjoining dendrites, they are released back into the synaptic cleft and reabsorbed by the host brain cell.

■ NEUROTRANSMITTERS

As a teacher, one has the tendency to pause and take a deep breath before continuing into a discussion of neurotransmitters. What are these brain cell messengers? How to explain something about which so little is known? Each year additional groups and subgroups of these electrochemical, or electrical, messengers are identified; and the systems in which they operate become more complex accordingly. At the same time, the effects of psychoactive drugs on these systems are seen as correspondingly more complex and more potentially dangerous to the user. A recent advertising campaign for drug abuse prevention used the image of an egg frying in a frying pan: "This is your brain on drugs." Ah, if only it were that simple.

A review of the current literature makes it clear that any detailed exposition of drug neurochemistry takes a perilous path through rapidly changing and often contradictory theories and paradigms. In that our primary concern in this book is that of providing useful information for the non-addiction-specialist, the authors will refrain from a detailed exposition of drug/brain neuro-chemistry—that could well be more than half obsolete with the next research breakthrough—and present instead a pastiche of general insights into this complex arena.

This is the User's Brain on Drugs:
A Neurochemistry of Opioid Analgesics

■ ENDOGENOUS OPIOIDS

The neurotransmitter system most directly involved in opioid analgesic use involves a family of endogenous pain control mes-sengers that include endorphins and enkephalins. Heroin and other opioids directly occupy receptor sites utilized by endorpins and enkephalins of the endogenous opioid system. Opioids also activate the dopamine neurons.

Since the early breakthroughs on addiction neurochemistry, it is now possible, with the exception of solvents, to construct speci-fic and testable hypotheses on the mechanisms of how most psy-choactive drugs work in the brain. The research breakthroughs began in the 1970s with the identification of endogenous mor-phines, better known as endorphins, within the brain. These endor-phines essentially turn off the pain-signal switch in the brain, bringing relief and even a feeling of well-being when they occupy specific receptor sites. It is now clear that at least three types of non-indigenous substances will also bind to these receptor sites. These are opioid agonists, partial agonists, and antagonists.

■ OPIOID AGONISTS

Nazi Germany almost discovered opioid neurotransmitters during World War II. Cut off from Near East opium supplies, Hitler's armies were without pain medication. German scientists were put on a crash program to develop a synthetic CNS analgesic that could be used in battlefield conditions, and what they came up with was methadone. Given that there were a number of priorities beyond pure science at the time, the German scientists were content with knowing that methadone worked for pain control without having to know why it worked. In retrospect, why it worked was that a part of the molecular structure of methadone was essentially the same as a part of the molecular structure of heroin and the endogenous morphines. Coincidentally, the part that coincided was the part that was needed to bind to the opioid receptor sites, but it took nearly 30 years to learn that truth about opioid receptors and ligands.

In the course of that research, it was determined that drug derived from opium and pain medications with a molecular structure similar to the opiates such as methadone and demerol had central nervous system effects similar to those attributed to endorphins and enkephalons. Some of the experiments involved the use of naloxone, an opioid receptor antagonist, a substance that had been used in emergency medicine to reverse the effects of opiate drug overdoses, in the reversing of endorphine effects as well.

■ OPIOID ANTAGONISTS

Up until that time, no one had understood how naloxone (Narcan®) worked. Only that it did work. As it became clear that opioids achieved their analgesic and other psychoactive effects by binding to endogenous morphine receptor sites, it also became clear that naloxone and other substances that came to be called opioid antagonists countered the effects of opioids by occupying and blocking the same receptor sites. Naloxone and the longer acting naltrexone had the ability to literally kick the opioid molecules out of the receptor sites and block their rebinding. As long as the opioid antagonists occupied the receptor sites, the opioid molecules were harmless, circulating in the bloodstream until they were metabolized and excreted.

The only exception to this process is when the overdose involves methadone or LAAM, two opioid "agonists," long-acting opioid receptor agonists that exert a narcotic depressant effect but are much longer acting. These substances will metabolize much more slowly than naloxone, and when the antagonist leaves the receptor sites will reoccupy them, thus reinstating the overdose. Given the possibility of a recurring overdose, the patient requires continued intravenous naloxone infusion to maintain the opioid receptor block until the long-acting drug has been metabolized.

■ OPIOID RECEPTORS

According to Jaffe and Jaffe,[4] there are three major types of opioid receptors, although additional types and sub-types have been proposed by researchers. Each of the major types has its own distinct distribution in the central and the peripheral nervous systems. Currently, over 20 pharmaceutical drugs act on the opioid receptors and generally produce analgesia, some form and degree of euphoria, decreased anxiety, respiratory, and cardiac suppression and a variety of other responses, including cough suppression for which heroin was originally prescribed and suppression of the limbic system in general.

When smoked or taken intravenously, the stronger opioids, such as morphine and heroin, which penetrate the brain rapidly, may produce a brief but intense sensation, a "rush" that has been described as a full body orgasm, followed by a "high," a longer lasting altered state characterized by disinhibition euphoria and a sense of detachment sometimes referred to as "being in a wicker basket." Often the individual nods in an opioid euphoria sleeplike state, feeling "no pain" until withdrawal starts as the drug wears off, and then panic sets in.

Sedative-Hypnotics

■ NEUROCHEMISTRY OF SEDATIVE-HYPNOTIC DRUGS

Sedative-hypnotic drugs are thought to achieve their primary effects through interacting with the gamma-aminobutyric acid

(GABA) neurotransmitter system. Studies on alcohol/brain inter-action are the most plentiful in that alcohol is the world's most pervasive sedative-hypnotic drug. It follows that the theories regarding alcohol and the brain have tended to be complex and contradictory.[5]

Since the reports of finding specific benzodiazepine-binding sites in the rat brain,[6,7] the character of the benzodiazepine recep-tor site has been the subject of intense research. These receptor sites, localized in synaptic contact regions in the cerebral cortex, cerebellum, and hippocampus, are associated with gamma-ami-nobutyric acid (GABA) receptor sites and affect their affinity for binding to a specific site, and also modify the cell membrane's per-meability to chloride ions. We have hypothesized that low-dose benzodiazepine withdrawal is receptor-site mediated.[8] A recep-tor-site-mediated withdrawal syndrome could plausibly explain why benzodiazepine withdrawal symptoms take more time to resolve than non-benzodiazepine sedative-hypnotic withdrawal symptoms.

Stimulants

■ NEUROCHEMISTRY OF STIMULANT DRUGS

It is generally agreed that cocaine has its neurochemical effects through activating the release of dopamine and blocking the re-uptake of synaptic dopamine. Cocaine also has an affinity for the serotonin binding sites and blocks the reuptake of both serotonin and the catecholamine norepinephrine. Amphetamine and methamphetamine have similar courses of action. As opposed to opioid analgesics and sedative-hypnotic drugs, which are post-synaptic drugs that bind directly to the neurotransmitter receptor sites, stimulant drugs are considered to be pre-synaptic. This means that they bind to sites within the brain that trigger the release of dopamine and norepinephrine, reinforcing stimulatory neurotransmitters. This overstimulation of the brain triggers the release of the inhibitory neurotransmitter serotonin. In much the same way that a jammed accelerator can burn out the brake when you try to control a car's speed by riding the brake, excessive stimulation can delete the brain's serotonin, leading to a post-stimulant crash with depression.

In blocking the reuptake of these neurotransmitters, stimulant drugs can create something like a chain reaction whereby the dopamine, serotonin, and norephinephrine continue to active sites in a number of cells until they are digested by enzymes that live between the brain cells and keep the spaces in the brain free of debris. These enzymes can be visualized as being like the early computer game "Pacman," i.e., traveling dots with mouths that eat everything in their path. The second effect of reuptake blocking is that the brain's supply of these neurotransmitters eventually decrease to the point where the stimulant drugs no longer have any effect. This depletion is dose-dependent and can be quite rapid for heavy users. Consequently, heavy stimulant use tends to be periodic, producing a binge behavior of use until the user's brain is incapable of supplying the key neurotransmitters. The use pattern that results is one of repeated binge/crash cycles, with a period of days or even weeks between binges while the user's brain replenishes supplies of the needed neurotransmitters. Once these have been replenished, the user experiences renewed drug hunger, i.e., the desire to use, and another binge ensues.[9]

Hallucinogens

■ A MULTIPLICITY OF AGENTS

Although they have been lumped together into a convenient category, hallucinogens do not represent a behaviorally homogeneous class of drugs. Glennon[10] separates hallucinogens into three general sub-categories, i.e., PCP-like psychotomimetics, cannabinoids, and cholinergic hallucinogens. Contingent with subclassification is the observation that these sub-categories produce their actions by differing neuropharmacological routes.

■ CLASSICAL HALLUCINOGENS VS. PCP

Classical hallucinogens, such as LSD and mescaline, are thought to act through serotonin 5-HT2 receptors. According to Glennon, hallucinogens can display widely varying binding profiles, however, the 5-HT2 receptor affinity is the one feature that they all have in common.

Phencyclidine (PCP) and its cogeners appear to have a route or routes of action that are quite different from those of classic hallucinogens. These may be highly complex in that PCP will produce very different effects depending upon dosage and bodily retention of the drugs, acting as stimulants at low dosage, depressants at mid-range dosages and mind–body dissociative hallucinogens at high dosages.

The Neuropharmacology of Marijuana

A very long-acting drug, marijuana has prominent effects on the central nervous system (CNS) and a number of peripheral effects. It is presently the most widely used illicit drug, particularly by young people, and is therefore worthy of a closer look.

While marijuana can be eaten, the most common mode of marijuana self-administration is by smoking and inhalation. Marijuana smoke contains more than 150 compounds in addition to the major psychoactive component, delta-9-tetrahydrocannabinol (THC). Many of the cannabinoids and other complex organic compounds appear to have psychoactive properties and others have not been tested for long- or short-term safety in animals or human beings.

The pharmacokinetics of marijuana is complex, starting with the volatilized THC produced by the burning of the cigarette, followed by the deep inhalation. Marijuana is rapidly absorbed from the lungs and THC and major metabolites can be traced throughout the body and brain. In the past, there had been some debate over whether marijuana's main constituent, THC, acts directly on the CNS or whether it must first be metabolized to 11-OH THC. It appears that THC is directly psychoactive.[11]

When marijuana is smoked, it appears to produce its psychoactive effects through specific binding with endogenous "THC" receptors. Radioligand binding studies with a water-soluble cannabinoid have revealed high-affinity sites in the brain that are specific for cannabinoids and that can be inhibited by myelin-basic protein in the rat.[12] Anandamide (the name given to the structure of arachidonylethanolamide, the brain's endogenous THC, an arachidonic acid derivative in the porcine brain) has recently been shown to inhibit the specific binding of a radiolabeled cannabinoid probe to synaptosomal membranes in a manner typical of competitive ligands. This effect produces a concentration-dependent inhibition of the electrically evoked twitch response of the mouse vas deferens, a characteristic effect of psychotropic cannabinoids. These properties suggest that anandamide may function as a natural ligand for the cannabinoid receptor.[13] In the first in vivo examination of anandamide, Fride and Mechoulam[14] reported that it produced hypothermia and analgesia, effects that parallel those caused by psychotropic cannabinoids. By defining the endogenous neurochemical process as with previous endogenous endorphin research, the identification of a THC receptor and its ligand helps to explain marijuana's analgesic, anti-nausea, concentration, and memory problems effects by showing that the drug has an affinity to areas in the brain involving pain and nausea control, and cerebral activities such as memory and concentration. Thomas and colleagues[15] reported that the cannabinoid binding of two ligands was densest in the basal ganglia and cerebellum (molecular layer), with intermediate binding in Layers I and VI of the cortex, and the dentate gyrus and CA- pyramidal cell regions of the hippocampus. The identification of a THC receptor and its ligand also suggests the possible development of new pharmacological treatments for marijuana abuse. Recent research with a THC receptor antagonist helps establish that cannabis dependence exists and may lead to a therapeutic agent, such as naltrexone, an opioid receptor antagonist agent which is both an opioid blocker and an anti-craving agent for alcohol.

Further verification of THC receptor has recently been announced by the American National Institute on Drug Abuse (NIDA).[16] Experiments involving the application of a THC antagonist, SR 141716A, produced a dramatic withdrawal syndrome in rats. According to senior investigator Billy Martin, M.D., "The fact that people do seek treatment for marijuana dependence is evidence of marijuana withdrawal in humans." Noting that withdrawal in humans is usually long and drawn out, he added, "But with rats, using SR 141716A as an effective antagonist, we compress and accentuate that withdrawal process."[17]

THC is highly lipid-soluble and a complex relationship exists between THC, which can be measured in the blood after self-administration, and rapid transfer into lipid and other areas of the central and peripheral nervous system. Direct correlations between self-reports of euphoria and blood levels have been hindered by this relationship and the metabolism of THC in the liver into 11-hydroxy-THC and 11-nor-carboxy THC[18] and tens of other metabolites with psychoactive properties. THC and THC metabolites are primarily excreted in the feces. The slow release of THC and active metabolites from lipid stores and other areas may explain the so-called carry-over effects on driving and other reports of behavioral changes over time. THC is stored in body fat and its slow excretion may make the urine test positive for more than 30 days, particularly if the individual is a chronic abuser. If the person is subject to drug testing in industry, the urine test can be positive, thereby putting the person's job in jeopardy, since the cut-off levels in industry are relatively low, i.e., 50 µg to 100 ng per mililiter. Even relatively low levels of use can be detected. This issue is further complicated by the fact that a prescription drug, Marinol (synthetic THC), used for glaucoma and the nausea associated with cancer chemotherapy, can make the urine screen positive for THC. In drug testing wherein an employee has been referred to the company's Employee Assistance Program for evaluation, including urinalysis, a medical review officer (MRO), usually a physician retained by the company to review all cases in which a potentially positive urine is reported, is necessary to make the distinction between medical use and illicit use.[19-21]

REFERENCES

1. Nutt DJ: The neurochemistry of addiction, in: Graham AW, Schultz TK, Wilford BB (eds.), *Principles of Addiction Medicine,* 2nd ed. Chevy Chase, MD: American Society of Addiction Medicine, 1998, p. 51.
2. National Institute on Drug Abuse: *The 1994 National Household Survey.* Chevy Chase, MD: National Institute on Drug Abuse, 1994.
3. Snyder SH: *Drugs and the Brain.* New York: Scientific American Library, 1986.
4. Jaffe JH, Jaffe AB: Neurobiology of opiates/opioids, in: Galanter M, Kleber HD (eds.), *Textbook of Substance Abuse Treatment,* 2nd ed. Washington, DC: American Psychiatric Press, Inc, 1999, p. 11.
5. Tabakoff B, Hoffman PL: Neurobiology of alcohol, in Galanter M, Kleber HD (eds.), *Textbook of Substance Abuse Treatment,* 2nd ed. Washington, DC: American Psychiatric Press, Inc, 1999, p. 3.
6. Mohler H, Okada T. Benzodiazepine receptors: demonstration in the central nervous system. *Science,* 1977; 198: 849–851.
7. Squires RF, Braestrup C: Benzodiazepine receptors in rat brain. *Nature,* 1977; 266: 732–734.
8. Wesson D, Smith, DE: Low dose benzodiazepine withdrawal syndrome: receptor site mediated. *California Society for the Treatment of Alcoholism and Other Drug Dependencies News,* 1982; 9: 1–5.
9. Fischman MW, Haney M: Neurobiology of stimulants, in: Galanter M, Kleber HD (eds.): *Textbook of Substance Abuse Treatment,* 2nd ed. Washington, DC: American Psychiatric Press, Inc, 1999, p. 21.
10. Glennon RA: Neurobiology of hallucinogens, in: Galanter M, Kleber HD (eds.), *Textbook of Substance Abuse Treatment,* 2nd ed. Washington, DC: American Psychiatric Press, Inc, 1999, p. 33.
11. Lemberger L, McMahon R, Archer R: The role of metabolic conversion on the mechanisms of action of cannabinoids, in Braude MS, Szara S (eds.), *Pharmacology of Marihuana,* Vol. 1. New York: Raven Press, 1976; 125–133.
12. Nye JS, McMahon R, Archer R: The role of metabolic conversion on the mechanisms of action of cannabinoids, in Braude MS, Szara S

(eds.), *Pharmacology of Marihuana*, Vol. 1. New York: Raven Press, 1976; 125–133.

13. DeVane WA, Hanu L, Bruer A: Isolation of a brain constituent that binds to the cannabinoid receptor. *Science*, 1992; 258: 1946–1949.

14. Fride E, Mechoulam R: Pharmacological activity of the cannabinoid receptor agonist anandamide, a brain constituent. *European Journal of Pharmacology*, 1993; 23(2): 313–314.

15. Thomas BF, Wei X, Martin BR: Characterization and autoradiographic localization of the cannabinoid binding site in rat brain using [3H]-OH-delta 9-THC-DMH. *Journal of Pharmacology and Experimental Research*, 1992; 263(3): 1383–1390.

16. Swan N: Marijuana antagonist reveals evidence of THC dependence in rats. *NIDA Notes*, 1995; 10(6): 1 & 6.

17. Aceto MD, Scates SM, Lowe JA, Martin BR: Cannabinoid-precipitated withdrawal by a selective antagonist: SR 141716A. *European Journal of Pharmacology,* 1995; 282(1–3): RI–R2.

18. Wall ME, Sadler BM, Brine D: Metabolism, disposition and kinetics of delta-9-tetrahydrocannabinol in men and women. *Clinical and Pharmacological Therapy*, 1983; 34: 352–363.

19. Seymour RB, Smith DE: Controlling substance abuse in the workplace, in: LaDou J (ed.), *Occupational Health and Safety,* 2nd Edition. Itasca, IL: National Safety Council, 1994; 287–306.

20. Seymour RB, Smith DE: Identifying and responding to drug abuse in the workplace. *Journal of Psychoactive Drugs*, 1990; 22(4): 383–405.

21. Clark HW: The medical review officer and workplace drug testing. *Journal of Psychoactive Drugs*, 1990; 22(4): 435–445.

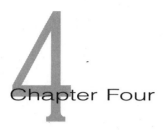

Chapter Four

The Signs and Symptoms of Abuse and Addiction

Addictive Disease and Denial

It is only in the most extreme of circumstances that the alcoholic or other drug addict will voluntarily seek treatment. In fellowships within the recovering community, such as Alcoholics and Narcotics Anonymous, it is well known that individuals who seek help for their addictions have generally "hit bottom." In other words, life has become so totally unbearable for them that they have no choice but to admit to themselves that their lives are out of control and something is drastically wrong.

Rather, practicing addicts who have not hit bottom or in some other way come face to face with their addiction in a forceful enough manner so as to break through their denial will stoutly maintain that there is no problem. At least they will maintain that the problem is not theirs. When pushed on the subject, they will maintain that their use is under control, they can quit any time; their families are mistaken or over-sensitive; after all, they are maintaining a steady job (if they still have one). How can they be addicts/alcoholics? Students of addictive disease have learned that this is not some form of intellectual stubbornness, nor is it conscious lying or manipulation on the part of the addict.

The Mid-brain Plot and its Co-conspirators................................

In Chapter 3, the authors pointed out that the seat of addiction is in the primitive mid-brain, below the level of intellectual consciousness. The seat of denial lies in the same territory. In essence, the addict is not consciously aware of his or her self-deception or addiction, for the primitive brain tells the thinking new brain that you must continue to use no matter what the consequences or you will not survive. This compulsive repetition can be described as reward reinforcement, which is a characteristic of all addicting drugs and is mediated through the dopamine pathways in the nucleus accumbens, which is part of the primitive brain. He or she is the victim of a conspiracy of silence, a web of secrecy created in the mid-brain and often supported by well meaning family, friends, and coworkers.

The web of silence is an aspect of what is called "codependence," wherein the individuals who are close to the addict: spouse, children, friends, etc., are drawn into a behavior pattern based on group denial that the addict has a problem. In recovering circles this is known as the "elephant in the living room syndrome." Everyone knows that the elephant is there, but everyone ignores it and works around it.

In professional circles, the dire consequences of discovery may contribute to a code of silence. This has been particularly true in the healing and law enforcement professions. One doctor who is now in long-term recovery and lectures on the nature of addiction and denial begins many of his presentations by hauling an extremely thick patient history to the podium where he reads excerpts:

- Patient brought in for observation after minor auto accident and released.
- Patient treated for cuts and abrasions after falling down from stairs and released.
- Patient resuscitated after becoming unconscious at dinner table.
- Patient treated for minor cuts after falling into Christmas tree, wife administered a mild sedative.

It goes on. And on. The doctor points out that the patient was a physician at the hospital where all the treatment described took place over a period of more than a decade. "During the same period, the physician attended many hospital social functions and had to be driven home from more than a few. More often, and worse, he drove home unchallenged even though he was in no condition to do so. In all that time, no colleague ever suggested that the physician might have a drinking problem. How do I know all this? Because I am that physician. Hello. My name is ＿＿ and I am an alcoholic."

Breaking Through the Conspiracy

How then, if the addict denies that there is a problem and everyone around the addict agrees that there is no problem, can the addict ever be identified? Should we all become coconspirators and banish the elephant from our collective consciousness. Should we let the addict continue to live in a dream world where nothing is wrong?

The answer is a resounding no. Addiction is a life-threatening disease that is toxic not only to the addict but to everyone with whom the addict comes into contact. When one considers that the addict could be a train engineer, an airline pilot, a surgeon, or even a cross-country truck driver, the potential danger becomes even more apparent. Beside the danger to themselves and others, addicts can also create a critical drain on the economy. The consequences of drug abuse and addiction, in terms of absenteeism, accidents, and the like, costs industry millions, perhaps billions of dollars every year.

Why Do People Use Drugs?

The personal consequences of drug abuse and addiction can include loss of dignity and self-worth, loss of job, loss of wife and family, possible imprisonment, enslavement to drugs and finally death at the hands of a progressive and potentially fatal disease. With so much at stake, why, one would ask, do people take the risk? Why do people use drugs? The motivation for drug use is varied and may change over time, even for the same drug and person. The following are four general categories of motivation.

■ PERFORMANCE FACILITATION

Some drug use is an attempt by the individual to work harder, or to be more productive, to increase energy in general, or to facilitate sexual activity. In the workplace, a piece worker may alternate amphetamines and opioids to increase the ability to work longer and faster and then turn it off without intolerable discomfort. Executives may use cocaine to help them work past their usual fatigue limit. Writers and other creative individuals may use alcohol or cocaine to facilitate or enhance their creative output.

■ RELIEF OF BOREDOM

Some jobs are inherently routine and offer only rare opportunity for challenge; others are structured to have a person available in case of equipment malfunction or in the event of an atypical condition. Even management of a household can be a stultifying series of repetitive tasks. With increasing automation, work and life may be less physically strenuous than in the past, but it has become more and more tedious. Maintenance drinking or using may protect the individual in such a plight from terminal boredom and is very hard to detect until such time as the out of the ordinary or emergency situation arises that requires peak alertness and rapid-judgment performance by the individual to avert disaster.

■ PROGRESSION INTO ADDICTION

What may have started out as experimentation or social use progresses from episodic, leisure-time use to chronic use, to loss of

control and continued use in spite of escalating adverse consequences.

■ SELF-MEDICATION

Individuals may self-medicate for a variety of reasons: to overcome shyness in social situations; to medicate a physical condition, such as tremors; to mediate chronic pain; even to counter
drug use symptoms, such as hangovers from alcohol or the jitters
from stimulant use.

Health Professionals: The First Line of Defense

In that alcohol and other drug addiction may develop slowly over
time, and in that all the individuals: family, friends, coworkers and
even employers may have become part of the addict's codepen-
dency web and as caught up in denial as the addict, an objective
health professional may well be the first line of defense in recognizing the presence of addiction. The addict may see a family doctor
routinely, or the encounter may be the result of a drug-related accident or mishap, or it may be an EAP (employee assistance program) referral for performance problems in the workplace.

Most companies have requirements for yearly physical examinations of their employees. Other individuals with private or
health maintenance organization (HMO) coverage may be
required to have periodic checkups. Such referrals and checkups
can provide an important opportunity for early detection and diagnosis of alcohol or other drug dependence. However, as the doctor
described at the beginning of this chapter discovered, physicians
may miss the opportunity to establish an early diagnosis of abuse
or addictive disease. This may happen for a number of reasons,
including:

1. Patient confidentiality is a tradition of medicine. Physicians
   may be ambivalent or uncertain about their role in the detection of conditions that their patients do not present as a prob-

lem. This issue can be particularly acute if reporting the condition could adversely affect the patient's employability—
even more acute if the patient happens to be a colleague.

2. In business referrals, physicians may perceive that management will not be appreciative of a diagnosis of alcohol or
other drug dependence because the diagnosis will require a
response by management with potential legal, union, and
employee grievance problems. Although some companies
provide health coverage for the treatment of alcohol and
other drug dependence, there is resistance to unqualified
acceptance of these disorders as diseases that could evoke
workers' compensation benefits.

3. Physicians may underdiagnose conditions that they believe
are medically untreatable. Many physicians who are not
addiction specialists do not view alcohol and other drug
dependence as a treatable illness. Physicians trained in public
institutions, where most alcohol and other drug-dependent
patients are often not motivated for treatment, develop pessi-
mistic attitudes regarding the treatability of such dependence.

4. Physicians may stereotype an alcoholic as a skid row derelict
and thus not consider the diagnosis of alcohol or other drug
dependence could possibly apply to working and more
respectable and affluent patients.

5. Physicians may have stereotypes of other drug users as street
people, "junkies" who are not employed in conventional jobs
or leading what may appear to be conventional lives.

6. Physicians may not inquire about alcohol and other drug use
for fear of evoking a response of indignant anger from their
patients.

7. Physicians without a specific interest in alcohol or other drug
dependence may not know about available laboratory screening procedures and may not recognize variations in a routine
laboratory test resulting from the compulsive use of alcohol
and other drugs. [1,2]

Until recently, and to some extent as a result of the legal fallout
from the 1914 Harrison Narcotic Act, which resulted in a progres-

sive court mandated separation of primary-care medical treatment of addiction in favor of a criminal justice approach to all drug problems, organized medicine maintained a firewall between itself and addiction treatment. This policy, engendered to place medicine above any suspicion of being a cause of iatrogenic addiction, was reflected in medical education.

Medical Education and Changing Standards of Practice

One of the top addiction medicine specialists received his medical degree and did post-doctoral work in toxicology at one of the leading west coast medical schools in the early 1960s. Throughout his course work, that physician had access to one class on addictive disease. That class was a Saturday afternoon elective presented by a recovering physician whose story appears in the Big Book of Alcoholics Anonymous.[3]

In the 1970s, in recognition of the growing drug problems, the federal government provided support for the Career Teachers in Substance Abuse program. That program supported the presentation of teachers and courses on substance abuse in a number of medical schools. The Career Teachers program lost its funding in the Reagan administration, but a number of the universities and teachers in the program stayed the course and continued aspects of the program.

Although standards of practice may have allowed physicians to ignore surreptitious alcohol and other drug dependence, the standard of practice as applied to drug abuse and addiction is changing. Attorneys are filing suits on behalf of clients injured by drug-impaired employees, against companies and against industrial physicians for failure to diagnose the drug-impaired condition. Major cases involving substance-related impairment, such as the *Exxon Valdez* case, have increased national concern. The disclosure of personal battles with alcohol and other drug dependence by such respected public figures as Betty Ford has helped break down stereotypes and has increased sympathy for individuals caught up in the disease of addiction. Finally, even though many practicing physicians and other health professionals did not receive training in recognizing and understanding substance abuse and addiction, means have been developed to make up for the deficit. Many states now require that health professionals enroll in a minimum amount of continuing medical education (CME) in order to maintain their license. Often a percentage of that CME is mandated to courses on substance abuse and addiction.

Today, a more enlightened medical community is working to break down the firewall between medicine and addiction. Steps are being taken to reverse some of the decisions of the 1920s and 1930s and give primary-care physicians and other health professionals a greater role in abuse and addiction treatment. A first step, however, is learning to detect the signs and symptoms and knowing what to do when they become apparent.

What the Health Professional Needs to Do—and Know.....

Examining physicians should routinely inquire about the use of alcohol and other drugs when they take a medical history. Early signs may be behavioral. For example, patients who are concerned about their abuse may deny use or minimize the amount used, but an emotional response to routine questions about drug use increases the probability of the patient having a substance abuse problem. An indirect question—such as, Is anyone in your family concerned about your alcohol (or other drug) use?—is a good screening question. Many drug users will acknowledge a family member's concern, followed by the reasons why the family member is wrong or doesn't understand.

Unless the patient's abuse is totally out of control, he or she will not come to a medical examination intoxicated, even on a day off work. Most alcoholics will make a point of not drinking for a day before their medical examination. (If they cannot control use even to that extent, they may call the doctor's office, or have an enabling codependent call for them, and cancel the appointment. Numerous canceled appointments may be a clue that something is wrong.) If they do comply and come in sober, abstinence may result in their being in a mild state of alcohol withdrawal with tremor, anxiety, increased pulse rate, increased blood pressure, and perspiration. Besides a thorough medical history and behavioral observation during the examination, information from work supervisors and/or family members and any history of unusual work or home injuries may suggest a diagnosis of alcohol or other drug dependence.

Arrests for driving under the influence are public record in many states and can be used to help confirm a diagnosis. An individual may unwisely drive once while intoxicated and learn by paying the penalties, but repeating the behavior after such adverse consequences may indicate that alcohol use is out of control.

Clues in Lab Work

Organ pathology and other physical manifestations can show up in lab tests. Hypertension can result from daily heavy drinking, and treatment of the hypertension is not effective unless the alcoholism is also treated. The most sensitive laboratory finding for alcoholism is an elevation of a liver enzyme, delta-glutamic transferase (GGT). Unless explained by liver disease unrelated to abuse or prescribed medication, such a phenobarbital, an elevated GGT in an otherwise healthy individual is presumptive evidence of advanced alcohol abuse. Another presumptive indicator of chronic alcohol abuse is an increase in red blood cell size that occurs as a result of alteration in folic acid metabolism. The average red blood cell size is usually measured in complete blood counts that are routine in physical examinations. Elevations of uric acid and triglycerides are also common in alcoholism, but may have other causes.

Observation as a Means of Early Detection...................

■ BEHAVIORAL SIGNS

Besides annual and other physical examinations, there are other means of identifying possible abuse and dependence. Working with health professionals, family, friends, and on the job supervisors and safety personnel can take a primary and direct role in pre-screening approaches by being aware of the behavioral signs of abuse and dependence.

Reports of the patient's behavior from spouse, friends, work supervisors or other individuals are an often effective type of behavioral assessment. Behavioral and psychological effects of alcohol and other drug abuse may include chronic tardiness or absenteeism at work, decreased performance and productivity, borrowing money from a number of sources, changes in mood or affect, and confusion.

Drug use sometimes causes no effects other than those produced shortly after the drug is taken; at other times, one or more effects can be seen chronically. In the first case, even the highly trained observer may not notice any effects unless the drug is detected by a urine or blood test. In the second case, the symptoms of drug use will sometimes resemble those of fatigue, a cold, stress and anxiety from problems at home or at work. Symptoms may not always be considered negative. For example, one early symptom of addiction—particularly to cocaine or other stimulant drugs—may be over-achievement, which serves to mask the actual problem. Even though the observed symptoms may not be drug related, unless they are the result of a transitory illness they do suggest that something is wrong and should be brought to the attention of a physician.

Behavioral signs may be most apparent in day to day activities in the home or in the workplace, or with adolescents in a school environment. Here are several categories that may indicate a problem.

Behavioral or Psychological Changes

The first adverse effect of substance use, abuse, or addiction is often a behavioral or psychological change. One of the most common indications is when an employee who has been punctual begins to repeatedly arrive late, or even misses days, often with no advance notice. When confronted with this behavior, the real cause is usually concealed, and the patient provides a justification that can be more or less convincing, particularly if backed up by an enabling codependent. Often a wife or husband will call an employer on the patient's behalf. In extreme cases, the reasons given for absence may be extremely imaginative. When stimulant psychosis is a factor, excuses may be increasingly bizarre and include such elements as kidnapping or brushes with the criminal underworld.

Decreased Productivity

Another sign is when patients stop taking interest in events at home or when employees exhibit decreased work productivity and do not perform as efficiently, quickly, or accurately as they have been in the past. A number of possible problems may be indicated, including such medical issues as diabetes, cardiovascular problems, or in older patients early onset dementia or other forms of diminished capacity. Any of these, however, should alert the need for further medical diagnosis.

Borrowing Money

A third sign of trouble is when the patient starts borrowing money from family, friends and coworkers, often with no good reason or bizarre reasons, and fails to pay it back promptly. If the individual has many friends—particularly if the relationship has been a long and close one—they may not seriously question such requests, even if the requests are unusual. After a substance abusing friend or coworker has been uncovered and friends begin to compare notes, it is not uncommon to discover that they have collectively loaned that person considerable amounts of money and not been repaid. This problem is especially common with abuse of cocaine, opioids, alcohol, and amphetamines.

Changes in Mood or Affect

This may take the form of mood swings from low to high and back to low, or the development of persistent mood states, such as depression, anxiety, anger, or paranoia. All drugs of abuse have profound effects on mood, and these effects wax and wane according to the person's tolerance, the dose taken, the frequency of use, and the duration of action of the drug. Most drug abusers or addicts go through frequent cycles of intoxication and withdrawal, often several times a day, that can produce frequent unexplained mood changes. Such changes are more likely to be seen in abusers and addicts than in recreational users, and are more often seen around paydays or after weekends. Certain drugs of abuse are associated with specific mood states or states of mental confusion. Cocaine and other stimulants produce paranoia and anger; persistent use of depressants, such as barbiturates or high doses of benzodiazepines produce depression; hallucinogens can produce lapses in concentration and memory and a range of very serious psychiatric disorders.

■ PHYSICAL SIGNS OF WHICH A HEALTH PROFESSIONAL SHOULD BE AWARE

In Chapter 2, the authors discussed the nature of the four drug groups and the symptoms of intoxication, overdose, and withdrawal. The outward manifestations of these symptoms may be observed as physical signs of abuse. Other physical effects of substance abuse may include skin lesions, infections, trouble with nose, sinuses or lungs, and difficulty with balance and coordination.

Some forms of drug abuse produce marked physical effects and produce visible lesions. Intravenous injection of drugs (such as opioids, cocaine, and amphetamines) causes puncture marks and produces scarred veins called tracks. These appear as long thin lines on the arms or legs and are usually purplish, reddish, or maroon. Generally, the darker and longer the track marks appear, the longer the history of drug use.

Drug infections often cause skin infections, resulting in circular reddish areas that are swollen and tender. Although not readily observable, infections can also travel to other areas of the body, such as the lungs or heart valves, where they can cause very serious problems that require hospitalization. One common illness in people who inject drugs is hepatitis. The presence of serum hepatitis, as opposed to infectious hepatitis, is always a reason to suspect drug abuse. Currently hepatitis C, which can progress without any visible symptoms for years, is being detected in increasing numbers of current and past injection drug users. Any individual who has ever injected drugs should be tested for Hepatitis C. Another disease that can be spread by needle use is of course HIV. Much more will be said about all these drug-related problems and diseases in Chapter 8.

Cocaine users often develop nose and throat problems due to irritation of these passages by inhaling or snorting cocaine. This may take the form of bloody nasal discharge, a runny nose, infections of the nose or sinuses, or frequent coughing. Runny nose can also result from histaminic discharges in heroin use, and coughing can be a sign of chronic tobacco use. Cocaine users will sometimes lose all sense of smell, and this symptom is usually a tip-off for cocaine abuse. Finally, a symptom suggestive of substance abuse or addiction is drowsiness and trouble with balance and coordination. This is commonly seen in people who are taking depressants, including alcohol or opioids, and can be very dangerous if one is driving or operating machinery.

■ THE EYES HAVE IT: PUPIL DIAMETER AND NYSTAGMUS

Pinned or Dilated Pupils

Two signs that often indicate active abuse when other symptoms are not readily identifiable are pupil diameter and nystagmus. The diameter of pupils is a useful, quick, presumptive indicator of recent opioid use. Normal pupils are between 3 and 2.0 mm in diameter; however, following opioid use the pupils are constricted to 1.0–2.0 ml and are commonly called pinned. Tolerance to pupillary constriction does not develop with continued opioid use, so pupillary constriction is a useful sign, even in daily users.

Pupil size is normally altered by the amount of ambient light, therefore the observation should be made under low-light conditions. Also, substantial variability exists in pupil size between individuals. After having once observed a person's pupil diameter under a low-light condition, later observations of a markedly constricted pupil under similar lighting is strong presumptive evidence of opioid use. Although opioid use is the most common reason for pinned pupils, medications used in the treatment of glaucoma (increased pressure inside the eye) will also produce marked pupillary constriction that persists under low-light conditions. In an opioid overdose producing unconsciousness, pupils may be dilated even though the overdose was due to opioids. Pupillary dilation during an opioid overdose occurs due to the lack of oxygen in the brain, which produces pupillary dilation overriding the pupillary constriction induced by the opioids.

Nystagmus

Horizontal nystagmus is the persistent 1.0–2.0 ml back-and-forth eye movements occurring at eye positions of extreme lateral gaze. It is another useful presumptive sign of drug intoxication and one that is often used by highway patrol officers in roadside checks. The movements are induced by asking the subject to hold his or her head in a fixed position while tracking a finger, pen or small flashlight. The object to be tracked is moved across the subject's visual field at a distance of 12–20 cm from the face.

Observation of nystagmus is facilitated if a light source diagonal to the subject's eyes reflects a small point of light from the white portion of the subject's eye. The eye movement has a quick component to the side of the gaze and a slow return movement toward the nose. Most people will have 1–3 cycles of nystagmus after the eyes are moved to the extreme lateral position but the movement stops. In individuals who are intoxicated with alcohol or other sedative-hypnotic drugs, the back-and-forth eye movements persist. Called sustained horizontal nystagmus, this eye movement is strong presumptive evidence for alcohol or other sedative-hypnotic intoxication. A similar disturbance in eye movements occurs in extreme vertical gaze (vertical nystagmus), which may include a component of slight rotation of the eyes called rotary nystagmus. Phencyclidine (PCP) intoxication produces severe disturbances in eye movements, and back-and-forth eye movements can occur even when the intoxicated person is looking straight ahead (central nystagmus). Sustained nystagmus is out of the person's voluntary control and is objective, reproducible, and strong presumptive evidence for alcohol, other sedative-hypnotic, or PCP intoxication.

Drug Testing

All of the above notwithstanding, there are often no overt signs of drug abuse that can be identified with any degree of assurance without further testing. Given the nature of denial, self-report is generally not forthcoming, and in situations where the abuser or addict can be a danger not only to his or her self but to others as well, it becomes imperative that an objective and even documentable evidence of use be obtained. As the United States, and western culture in general, shifted from having a drug-abusing subculture to being a culture that frequently abused drugs, the need become even more critical.

In the 1980s, when industry and the American military became aware of the costs of drug addiction, they decided to deal with the problem as rapidly and efficiently as they could. Their goal was to identify, and eliminate drug addicts and abusers before they could do any further harm. The technology that presented itself for accomplishing the task was urine testing.[1,2]

In 1986, then-president Reagan signed into law the Federal Drug Free Workplace act, intended to serve as a national model for eliminating drug abuse within the labor force. A major component of this initiative was pre-employment, random, and probable-cause drug testing for what has become known as the "NIDA-5," marijuana, cocaine, amphetamine, opioids, and phencyclidine. The opposition to testing, particularly pre-employment and random testing has been intense, resulting in legal challenges that extended all the way to the United States Supreme Court, which upheld government drug testing for US Customs agents as well as railroad employees involved in accidents or safety violations.

The basis for legal support of drug testing has been that the government's interest in preventing drug use and ensuring the safety of the nation's transportation outweighs the employees' right to privacy. Such legal decisions in the public sector set the stage for more aggressive drug testing procedures in the private sector, advanced with general public support as a result of the widespread concerns about drug abuse in society.

Even though the government, the public, and industry generally supported drug testing, there has been substantial opposition to random drug testing in the workplace. The American Federation of State, County, and Municipal Employees argued, for example, that drug testing is a far more pervasive intrusion into personal privacy than any suspicionless search the court has ever validated, and stressed that the rights of many employees will be violated. Further, specialists in addiction medicine voiced concern that the focus of the drug-free workplace is primarily on illicit drugs, despite the fact that alcohol is the most prevalent drug causing work-related accidents. It has been estimated that alcohol contributes to over 100,000 deaths per year and costs society over $100 billion annually in health care, absenteeism, and lost productivity. Furthermore, nicotine, another legal drug, probably contributes to more than 400,000 deaths per year and costs society an additional $60 to $100 billion annually in health care, absenteeism, and lost productivity.

Two additional problems soon became evident in the rush to clean house on the basis of random drug screens. First, there were no clear guidelines for administering urine screens, processing the samples, or assessing the results. Companies with an eye on the bottom dollar were inclined to enlist the simplest and cheapest screen processes. Use of these and the frequency of less than ideal lab procedures produced questionable results, including false positives and negatives. Second, and compounding the technical problems, was the fact that many companies and government entities made positive drug tests the basis for draconian responses, including immediate dismissal and punitive responses. In the military, a positive drug screen was grounds for courts martial, incarceration, and dishonorable discharge. In the business world, summary firing, even of long-term employees could be the result of a positive screen. Lawsuits ensued, often on investigation settled in favor of the employee.

■ THE MISUSE AND ABUSE OF URINE SCREENS

Urine screens, properly used, can be a valuable diagnostic tool for confirming abuse, or in a treatment setting, for helping maintain treatment compliance. The problem in the 1980s was that the tool was being misunderstood, misused, and abused. Without critical analysis of just what a screen represented, serious mistakes effecting peoples' lives could occur. Besides false positives resulting from faulty lab procedures, there can be a variety of circumstances involved in what appears to be a positive screen that do not indicate drug abuse or addiction. With many of the mass screening processes, legitimate prescription drugs and some foodstuffs, such as poppy seeds, may show up as illicit drugs. Environmental factors may need to be taken into consideration.

In one example, during the period when military units were undergoing random urine testing, one of the authors received a phone call from a military police unit commander whose unit had been tested. One of his men had tested positive for marijuana and he was totally mystified. He described the man as a middle-aged non-commissioned officer with a spotless military record, a family man, a real straight arrow. It turned out that one of the sergeant's duties was disposing of confiscated marijuana that had been used as evidence in courts martial. He burned the material in an open base furnace provided for that purpose. What was needed was not just efficient drug screening but a means of interpreting the results.

■ PLACING URINE SCREENS IN CONTEXT AS A USEFUL DIAGNOSTIC TOOL

Several things have been done to bring drug screening into line with acceptable standards of diagnostic practice. These have involved not only the way screens are initiated and processed but what is done with the information obtained as well.

Testing Procedures

Procedurally, all supposedly positive tests now must be confirmed by a second procedure. Most laboratories use a screening test that attempts to identify a variety of drugs of abuse. This is a general test designed to detect the presence of a class of drugs. Because its aims are so general, it cannot be trusted to confirm the presence of a specific drug. This is also the type of screen that was most often employed by itself in military, school and workplace random drug screenings in the 1980s. Today, a specimen that is positive on this general screening test must be evaluated by a second procedure that uses a more specialized test directed at a particular drug.

The initial test used by many laboratories is known as thin-layer chromatography (TLC). Radioimmunoassay (RIA), Enzyme-multiplied immunoassay technique (EMIT), and fluorescence polarization immunoassay (FPIA) are other tests commonly used to screen for abusable drugs. Helpful as initial screens may be, they are far from perfect. A recent comparison showed discrepancies on false positives and false negatives even under the best of both screen application and laboratory conditions.[4] The confirmatory test most commonly accepted is gas chromatography-mass spectroscopy (GC-MS), which is generally considered to be a highly specific and accurate urine-testing technology.

Forensic Standards

Besides verification of test results, forensic standards have been developed for sample collection and handling. The transfer of urine, blood, or saliva from subjects to containers must be witnessed. If an individual is taken to a physician for the collection of a blood sample, the physician becomes the first link in the chain of custody, and consequently he or she must be instructed in and follow the requirements of legal chain-of-custody procedures. The observer must verify the accuracy of the container label (including the subject's name and other identifying information, date, time of collection, and type of collection receptacle) and must maintain the chain of custody of the sample until it reaches the laboratory.

Even with testing verification and forensic safeguards, tests need to be seen as existing within a context that may have bearing on the testing results. In recognition of this context, a screen is not officially positive until the case has been reviewed by a licensed physician with clinical experience in the field of industrial medicine, drug and alcohol abuse treatment programs, or drug testing programs and has a working knowledge of substance abuse disorders, medical use of prescription drugs, and the pharmacology and toxicology of illicit drugs. This medical review officer (MRO) agrees to review and interpret positive urine test results and present his or her findings. The review may be a complex procedure involving interviews with the subject, review of pertinent medical records, discussion with individuals involved in the collection, transport and analysis of the specimen, possibly re-testing of the same sample via a portion reserved and preserved for that eventuality, and discussions with the scientific director or a forensic toxicologist with the NIDA-certified laboratory that performed the test. Sometimes the most decisive factor may be finding out that the subjects duties include contact with burning cannabis. If after review the MRO determines that there is a legitimate medical explanation for the positive test result, the MRO reports the test result as a negative.

Urine, blood, breath, saliva, and even hair testing can play a role in the identifying and diagnosis of drug abuse and dependence. That role however, needs to be in context and part of an overall diagnostic process, and not as a free-standing indictment of the testee. Testing can also be helpful in verifying compliance during treatment, but it should never, in and of itself be used as grounds for expelling someone from a treatment program. One must keep in mind that addiction is a chronic disease characterized in part by frequent slips and relapses. Treatment is a window of opportunity in the task of moving a patient from active addiction to active recovery. Drug testing can be used to monitor the progress of this transition from active addiction to recovery and when relapse occurs, treatment can be adjusted accordingly. It should also be stressed that 100% of active alcoholics and addicts will surface at some time in the medical system, but only 5–10% end up in treatment for their addictive disease. Improved diagnostic testing can increase the number who go from medical complications of their disease to recovery from this potentially fatal illness.

REFERENCES

1. Seymour RB, Smith DE: Controlling substance abuse in the workplace, in: LaDou J (ed.), *Occupational Health and Safety*, 2nd ed. Itasca, IL: 1994, pp. 287–306.
2. Seymour RB, Smith DE: Identifying and responding to drug abuse in the workplace. *Journal of Psychoactive Drugs*, 1990; 22(4): 383–405.
3. Anonymous: *Alcoholics Anonymous: The Story of How Many Thousands of Men and Women have Recovered from Alcoholism*, 3rd ed. New York: Alcoholics Anonymous World Services, Inc., 1976.
4. Schilling RF, Bidassie B, El-Bassel N: Detecting cocaine and opioids in the urine: comparing three commercial assays. *Journal of Psychoactive Drugs*, 1999; 31(3): 305–313.

5

Chapter Five

Diagnosis and Assessment (DSM IV, SCID, and Other Criteria)

Diagnosis and assessment of substance abuse and addiction involves a number of variables. A clear understanding of which drug or drugs may be included in a complex polydrug abuse syndrome may well be a matter of life and death. Individuals at some levels of abuse or addiction can safely be detoxified on an outpatient or in a non-medical, social model setting. Others may be subject to potentially life-threatening withdrawal symptoms, such as grand mal seizures, if proper medical procedures are not followed. In a larger sense, it has become increasingly clear that addiction treatment, in order to be effective and long-lasting, needs to be diagnosis driven. There is no "one size fits all" approach to drug treatment. Therefore, it is of utmost importance that diagnosis and assessment in preparation for the treatment best suited to the individual patient be carefully and thoroughly undertaken.

Diagnosis-driven treatment means that the individuals treatment is tailored to the specific addiction syndrome and life situation of the individual patient. Does the patient need to be in a residential unit or will a day program serve as well? Is medical intervention necessary? Will a social model program, or a therapeutic community suffice? What are the particular ramifications of the drugs involved in the patient's use and which should be detoxified first? Are there psychiatric symptoms independent of the addiction? All these questions and many more need to be considered. In this chapter we will discuss some of the diagnostic and assessment tools in current use in addiction medicine. In the next chapter, we will move on to the varieties of treatment.

American Society of Addiction Medicine Patient Placement Criteria..

The patient placement criteria developed by the American Society of Addiction Medicine (ASAM)—see Appendix I—is probably the most significant current development in establishing a single, standardized set of criteria for matching patients to treatment. For that reason, the authors have included these criteria within this book. According to Gastfriend and colleagues[1] the ASAM criteria utilize four major levels of care: hospital, non-hospital, inpatient, day treatment, and outpatient; and includes a range of intensities of service within each of these principal levels of care. The criteria rely on six dimensions approach to assessment that takes into account a full range of clinical variables relevant to the matching process. These dimensions or problem areas are:

1. Acute intoxication and/or withdrawal potential.
2. Biomedical conditions and complications.
3. Emotional/behavioral conditions and complications.
4. Treatment acceptance/resistance.
5. Relapse/continued use potential
6. Recovery/living environment.

■ DIAGNOSIS-DRIVEN TREATMENT

The above considerations create the necessity for new approaches to clinical assessment and documentation. Patient records that traditionally served only to communicate clinical data among providers now becomes crucial in determining not only what type of care is needed but whether treatment is necessary. In an age of HMO justification, patient evaluations documenting an objective assessment process are needed to provide justification for any treatment recommendations. What develops is a system of treatment that is driven by a detailed diagnosis rather than by non-treatment-related considerations. This process may prove in the long term the most effective means to initiating cost-efficient, and clinically successful treatment.

■ THE USE OF DSM-IV IN CLINICAL DIAGNOSIS

According to Gastfriend and colleagues,[1] clinical diagnosis is probably the most fully developed assessment area, given the general acceptance of the *Diagnostic and Statistical Manual of Mental Disorders of the American Psychiatric Association* or *DSM-IV* criteria.[2] Several clinical interview instruments have been developed that can help establish a DSM-IV drug abuse disorder diagnosis, and of these the Structured Clinical Interview for DSM-IV (SCID)[3] is considered the most easily incorporated into a diagnosis battery for clinical evaluation.

SCID is a semi-structured interview designed for use with psychiatric, medical or community-based normal adults that can obtain Axis I and Axis II diagnoses on the basis of DSM-IV criteria. The interview was designed to be administered by master's or doctoral level trained clinical evaluators but has been used by BA level personnel with extensive training. Modules of the SCID are designed to address each of the major DSM-IV syndromes: anxiety disorder, affective disorders, psychotic disorders, and substance use disorders. The evaluation of possible dual diagnosis patients with Axis I and Axis II batteries may take over 2 hours, while administration of the Psychoactive Substance Use Disorders module on its own may take 30–60 minutes. The module, which encompasses questions based on abuse/dependence DSM-IV criteria for alcohol and each of the other psychoactive substances, can establish lifetime diagnoses, age of first abuse or dependence onset and current severity of the problem.

Other instruments currently in use include the Schedule for Affective Disorders and Schizophrenia (SADS)[4] and the Diagnostic Interview Schedule (DIS).[5] Both instruments have some drawbacks, as pointed out by Gastfriend and colleagues.[1]

SADS "... requires interviewers with graduate degrees and fairly extensive clinical experience and can take up to 4 hours to administer." DIS "... was designed for administration by non-clinicians and proceeds on a symptom-by-symptom basis, with the requirement that each question be read verbatim from a booklet.

Diagnostic and Statistical Manual of Mental Disorders, 4th Edition

In the manual much of the evaluative instruments are based on the DSM-IV, it behooves us to examine the criteria for substance dependence presented by that manual. The DSM-IV, as the edition number implies, is the latest in a series of diagnostic manuals developed and produced by the American Psychiatric Association. In the process of development since the first *Diagnostic and Statistical Manual* appeared in 1952, the criteria for drug dependence has undergone a series of evolutionary changes. In that first edition, alcoholism and drug addiction were classified within the category of "Sociopathic Personality Disturbances." By the second edition, in 1967, they fell under the broader designation of "Personality Disorders," and included such diagnostic terms as "dependence, abuse, addiction, and habitual use." In the 1980, third edition, definitions became less ambiguous and included specific criteria for diagnosing the disorders. Dependence was distinguished from abuse by the presence of tolerance and/or existence of a withdrawal syndrome. The 1987 revision, DSM-IIIR, de-emphasized physical aspects and recognized the variability of tolerance and withdrawal across different individuals and drugs. In that edition, Psychoactive Substance Dependence could be a diagnosis if the patient met any three of nine criteria:

1. tolerance;
2. withdrawal;
3. withdrawal avoidance;

4. socially dysfunctional use;
5. use despite problems;
6. cannot stop;
7. salience;
8. pre-occupation, and
9. cannot limit use.[6,7]

The DSM-IV goes into much more detail. Substance abuse is defined as a maladaptive pattern of substance use characterized by hazardous or compulsive use or the presence of role impairment or recurrent legal problems, but without evidence of tolerance or withdrawal. According to Ball and Kosten,[6] most individuals who meet the criteria for substance abuse and continue to use eventually will meet the criteria for dependence, laid out within the DSM-IV as follows.

■ DSM-IV CRITERIA FOR SUBSTANCE DEPENDENCE

Substance dependence is a maladaptive pattern of substance use, leading to clinically significant impairment or distress, as manifested by three (or more) of the following:

1. Tolerance, as defined by either of the following:

   (a) a need for markedly increased amounts of the substance to achieve intoxication or desired effect, or
   (b) markedly diminished effect with continued use of the same amount of the substance.

2. Withdrawal, as manifested by either of the following:

   (a) the characteristic withdrawal syndrome for the substance (refer to criteria A and B of the criteria sets for withdrawal from the specific substances), or
   (b) the same (or closely related) substance is taken to relieve or avoid withdrawal symptoms.

3. The substance is taken in larger amounts or over a longer period than was intended.

4. There is a persistent desire or unsuccessful efforts to cut down or control substance use.
5. A great deal of time is spent in activities necessary to obtain the substance (e.g., visiting multiple doctors or driving long distances), use of the substance (e.g., chain smoking), or recover from its effects.
6. Important social, occupational, or recreational activities given up or reduced because of substance use.
7. The substance use is continued despite knowledge of having a persistent or recurrent physical or psychological problem that is likely to have been caused or exacerbated by the substance (e.g., current cocaine use despite recognition of cocaine-induced depression, or continued drinking despite recognition that an ulcer was made worse by alcohol consumption).

Specify if:

> *With Physiological Dependence*: Evidence of tolerance or withdrawal (i.e., item 1 or 2 is present); or *Without Physiological Dependence*: No evidence of tolerance or withdrawal (i.e., neither item 1 nor 2 is present.[2]

■ ASSESSMENT OF DUAL DIAGNOSIS PATIENTS

Many substance abuse patients, up to 40% at the Haight Ashbury Free Clinics, also have psychiatric problems. Quite often, these patients require tandem treatment for both addiction and psychopathology. Diagnosing psychopathology in addicted individuals can, however, be a difficult proposition.

First, there is the difficulty of separating certain symptoms of drug abuse from those of primary psychiatric disorders. Foremost among these is the fact that many symptoms of active abuse and addiction are similar to those of psychiatric disorders. Chronic and intense abuse of stimulant drugs, for example, may produce a stimulant psychosis characterized by paranoia with ideas of reference as well as delusional states replete with hallucinations, known in the street as "tweaking."

Darryl Inaba, director of the Haight Ashbury Free Clinics drug treatment division, recommends writing any psychiatric assessment of a patient in the process of withdrawing and early recovery in disappearing ink.[8] At the minimum, a psychiatric assessment should not be attempted until the patient is no longer intoxicated and mood and cognitive status have had a chance to stabilize. A delay of 2–4 weeks into abstinence is preferable, but with severely addicted individuals at least 3–10 days with a concomitant mental status examination for adequate memory and concentration may be enough for an accurate assessment of the onset, course, and symptoms of a presumed psychiatric disorder.[9]

Primary drug effects that may mimic psychiatric disorders may take varying lengths of time to clear. The effects of phencyclidine (PCP), a drug that can remain active in the system for extended periods, were thought to be evidence of permanent brain damage until long-term abstinence in some PCP users proved otherwise. In general, the disorders related to addiction were until recently so prevalent that addiction was often considered a symptom of underlying psychosis. The disease concept of addiction, however, holds that it is a disease entity in and of itself with its own baggage of symptoms that begin to clear in time with a program of abstinence and supported recovery. The facts that drug abusers and addicts do often suffer from psychiatric disorders as well, that even though little headway can be made on treating such disorders as long as the patient is actively abusing alcohol or other drugs, that many individuals may be self-medicating for their psychiatric problems, all tell us that once ascertained both addiction and psychiatric disorders should be treated at the same time.

■ UTILIZING COLLATERAL INFORMATION

In situations where an accurate and rapid diagnosis is needed, collateral information can be utilized. Several systems have been developed to facilitate dual diagnosis or comorbidity diagnosis. These are the Best Estimate procedure[10] and the LEAD standard procedure.[11] Best Estimate involves expert review of the blinded records of structured interviews and collateral information from medical records and one or more interviews with the patient's family members. LEAD (Longitudinal, Expert diagnoses based on All available Data) involves administering the following:

- a comprehensive battery of assessments of psychiatric and addiction symptoms by a research associate within the first week of hospitalization, repeated approximately 2 weeks later by a psychiatrist;
- interviews with significant others about the patient's alcohol and drug use and psychiatric history;
- gathering of diagnostic information from other clinical staff by the psychiatrist at the patient's discharge conference; and
- review of recent and old chart information.

Such a procedure can be effective, particularly for diagnosing substance abuse disorders, but in most cases may be neither necessary nor cost-efficient. Diagnostic use of blood, urine, breath, or hair sample screens can provide a profile of the patients drug use status, while a physical workup can provide information on any long-term abuse sequelae. If there is any doubt as to the presence of comorbidity, observation should be continued until it is reasonable to assume that drug-generated symptoms would have cleared.

REFERENCES

1. Gastfriend DR, Baker SL, Najavits LM, Reif S: Assessment instruments, in: Graham AW, Schultz TK, Wilford BB (eds.), *Principles of Addiction Medicine,* 2nd ed. Chevy Chase, MD: American Society of Addiction Medicine, 1998, p. 273.
2. American Psychiatric Association: *Diagnostic and Statistical Manual of Mental Disorders,* 4th ed. Washington, DC: American Psychiatric Press, 1994.
3. First M, Gibbon M, Spitzer R, Williams J: *User's Guide for the Structured Clinical Interview for DSM-IV Axis I Disorders, Research*

Version (SCIDI, Version 2.0, February 1996). New York: Biometrics Research Department, New York State Psychiatric Institute.

4. Endicott J, Spitzer RL: A diagnostic interview: the schedule for affective disorders and schizophrenia. *Archives of General Psychiatry*, 1978; 35(7): 837–44.

5. Robins LN, Helzer JE, Croughan J, Ratcliff KS: National Institute of Mental Health diagnostic interview schedule. *Archives of General Psychiatry*, 1981; 38(4): 381–89.

6. Ball SA, Kosten TA: Diagnostic classification systems, in: Graham AW, Schultz TK, Wilford BB (eds.), *Principles of Addiction Medicine,* 2nd ed. Chevy Chase, MD: American Society of Addiction Medicine, 1998, p. 279.

7. American Psychiatric Association: *Diagnostic and Statistical Manual of Mental Disorders (I:* 1952; *II,* 1967; *III,* 1980; *IIIR,* 1987) Washington, DC: American Psychiatric Press.

8. Inaba D: Personal communication.

9. Rounsaville BJ, Kranzler HR: DSM-III-R diagnosis of alcoholism, in: Tasman A, Hale RE, Frances AJ (eds.), *Psychiatric Updates.* Washington, DC: American Psychiatric Press, 1989.

10. Leckman JF, Sholomskas D, Thompson WD, Belanger A, Weissman MM: Best estimates of lifetime psychiatric diagnosis: a methodological study. *Archives of General Psychiatry,* 1982; 39: 879–83.

11. Spitzer RL: Psychiatric diagnoses: are clinicians still necessary? *Comprehensive Psychiatry,* 1983; 24: 399–411.

Chapter Six

Abuse and Addiction Treatment: Treatment as the Bridge Between Active Addiction and Active Recovery

PART 1: TREATMENT OF ACUTE TOXICITY AND WITHDRAWAL

The Myths About Treatment

The treatment of alcoholism and other substance addictions suffers from two dominant but conflicting myths. On the one hand, many health professionals and much of the general public is convinced that attempting to treat addiction is a patent waste of time because addiction is incurable and no matter what is done, the addict will always return to active addiction. On the other hand there is a tendency for most physicians and for the general public to also perceive addictions as acute conditions, such as a broken leg or pneumococcal pneumonia.[1] How such contradictory views can be held, often by the same people at the same time, is a mystery. They do represent, however, myths that need to be dislodged if there is to be social, public health and medical progress in the treatment of addiction.

■ MYTH 1: THE ADDICT IS UNTREATABLE AND INCURABLE

The first of these myths, that addiction is essentially untreatable, grew in part out of the criminal justice system approach to addiction that was taken in the first half or so of the 20th century. Before the passage of the Harrison Narcotic Act in 1919, both opium and cocaine were easily available and had become prime ingredients in many forms of patent medicine. Their use in tonics and elixirs was so pervasive that at the turn of the century the typical opioid dependent could be characterized as a middle-aged, middle-class white woman with children.

Treatment for both opioid and cocaine addiction was largely a private matter and in the hands of physicians. There were dozens of theories for the treatment of addicts. According to Musto,[2] patients could be purged or sedated during withdrawal with a variety of substances including bromides, barbiturates, trional, etc., or put into a state of forgetfulness with hyoscine or atropine. Another drug, thought to be less harmful than the addict's drug of choice could be substituted and maintained. For example, heroin started out as a "cure" for morphine addiction. At the turn of the century, there was much confidence that addiction was eminently curable and dozens of sanitaria for alcohol and drug habits, mostly catering to wealthy and upper-middle-class clients, sprang up across the United States. By the 1920s, however, much of the confidence in rapid cure by detoxification had faded and substitution and maintenance with an alternative opioid or with cocaine was the most prevalent treatment. The pervading theory was that addicts' prolonged use had altered their chemistry so that the drug of choice, or drugs in the same family needed to be maintained on an ongoing basis.

At the same time, national attitudes toward addiction were undergoing a basic change. According to Musto, "In the post-World War I hysteria, however, attitudes changed. If outpatient treatment could not control deviance, if medical institutions like hospitals could not cure it, then police and jails were the last option."[2] The Harrison Narcotic Act was the first national law opening the door to control of "narcotics," defined as opioids and cocaine. In the following decade a series of court actions taken with the tacit support of organized medicine, which saw treatment of addiction as a threat to its relatively new but precarious state of respectability, the medical treatment of addiction was essentially criminalized and addiction treatment facilities were progressively shut down. Capping this process was a Supreme Court ruling that found the medical maintenance of an addict to be illegal.

By the 1930s, treatment of addiction had become a criminal justice matter. Treatment at the Lexington and Fort Worth Narcotic Hospitals was a procedure of maintaining addicts in locked wards while they endured an essentially "cold turkey" withdrawal. Cold turkey referred to withdrawal without medical intervention, and referred specifically to piloerection or goose bumps, one of the frequent symptoms of opioid withdrawal. The form of treatment adopted by the criminal justice system tended to provide an excruciating episode of enforced withdrawal but did nothing to alleviate the addict's addiction. As a consequence, a frequent first stop—or soon thereafter—when the addict was released was to the addict's dealer. A United States Public Health Service study in 1942 showed that over 75% of the addicts treated at the Lexington Narcotic Hospital relapsed soon after treatment, while a 1962 follow-up study indicated that 90% of the Lexington patients returning to New York were relapsing.[3]

The obvious extent of recidivism from these prison hospitals established an opinion within the law enforcement community that narcotic addicts were incurable. That opinion was reinforced for the general public with the appearance of Otto Preminger's film *The Man with the Golden Arm* in 1955. The unforgettable performance of Frank Sinatra as the hopelessly addicted gambler Johnny Machine solidified a nation's growing stereotype of the narcotic addict as an incurable low-life. Although the medical community had little to do with opioid or cocaine addicts in this period, health professionals tended to see a stereotyped version of the alcoholic as an equally incurable case.

■ MYTH 2: THE ADDICT CAN BE DETOXIFIED AND LIVE HAPPILY EVER AFTER

The element of truth behind Myth 1 is that addictive disease is chronic and the addict subject to slips and relapses. The chronic nature of the disease also is why the second myth, that addiction can be easily cured, is indeed a myth. There are very few addicts who can walk away at the end of a short-term program of detoxification and stay abstinent for a year, much less the rest of their lives. In truth, within the recovering community, the very concept that addiction can be cured is considered absurd on the face of it. There, the alcoholic or other addict is always recovering, never recovered, never cured. Recovery is considered to be a lifelong process.

The Reality of Treatment

The treatment of drug abuse and addiction includes three phases: emergency treatment for acute adverse reactions, overdose, or acute withdrawal; detoxification and aftercare; and long-term medical and behavioral therapy.

■ EMERGENCIES: OVERDOSE AND ACUTE WITHDRAWAL

The first stage of alcohol and other drug treatment is essentially emergency treatment for acute conditions. These conditions include opioid and sedative hypnotic (including alcohol) overdoses, acute adverse physical and mental reactions to hallucinogens, and stimulant drugs. Many acute drug reactions can be life-threatening, potentially fatal if not treated quickly. Often an emergency situation may be the first warning that there is a drug problem. Treated properly, emergency treatment situations may provide a window for initiating the patient into more comprehensive treatment for his or her drug problem. Drug emergencies may occur in the home and result in the patient being treated on site by a mobile unit following a 911 call, or being taken to an emergency room, hospital, clinic, or poison center. For young people, drug emergencies may occur at rock concerts or raves where it is to be hoped that alert field medics will intervene and convince them that they should seek further treatment. Youth gatherings are focal points at which drug initiation can take place, and as such provide a point where a young person's drug problems may begin to be addressed while they are still in an early stage of development.

■ ALL DRUGS ARE POISONS

All psychoactive drugs are poisons. At some level, each one of them becomes toxic to the human system and their presence in any quantity beyond that point becomes life-threatening. The emergency treatment of psychoactive drug poisoning falls within the medical science of toxicology, the study of toxic substances.

Effective medical response can differ greatly between the drug groups and so it can be of utmost importance to quickly identify at least what family of drug the patient has ingested. Lacking a clear reading of what drug or drugs may be involved, a diagnosis must be quick and sure. Particularly with opioid and sedative-hypnotic overdose, a quick response can be a matter of life and death.

■ OPIOID INTOXICATION AND OVERDOSE

Mild intoxication is characterized by euphoria and/or sedation. In severe intoxication and overdose, the causative interactions are with the mu opioid receptors in the central nervous system (CNS). These interactions can bring about both sedation and respiratory depression resulting from direct suppression of the respiratory centers in the brain stem and the medulla. O'Connor and Kosten[4] recommend a careful collection of patient data through history and physical examination while at the same time initiating pharmacological and supportive therapies to ameliorate morbidity and prevent mortality in patients with moderate to severe respiratory depression. Information concerning drug use can be elicited directly from the patient, if still conscious and coherent, from friends and/or family members and from hospital records if available. If possible, the information should include the drug or drugs that the patient has taken, how much and when taken. If the patient has taken more than one drug, such as a benzodiazepine or large amounts of alcohol at the same time as the opioid, additional therapies may need to be employed to reverse the other components.

A physical examination of the patient may show both CNS and respiratory depression, pinpoint pupils and such physical evidence of use as needle tracks or soft tissue infection. A urine toxicology screening can help rule out other possible causes of observed symptoms, such as hypoglycemia, acidemia, fluid and electrolyte abnormalities. Even though the screening results will probably not be available until after the initiation of acute management, they will help to suggest any modifications that may be called for and are a good means of ascertaining if any other drugs are involved and provide data for post-emergency treatment.

While the three physical symptoms of respiratory depression, coma and pinpoint pupils will alert treatment personnel to a potential opioid overdose, clinicians must be alert to atypical presentations. Whipple and colleagues point out that in a study of 43 patients hospitalized with suspected opioid overdoses, only two had presented with the above three symptoms.[5] The most telling means of diagnosis, however, lies in the patient's reaction to the specific pharmacologic therapy for opioid overdose, naloxone hydrochloride. If the patient does not respond to multiple doses of naloxone, alternate diagnoses should be considered.

■ NALOXONE HYDROCHLORIDE (NARCAN®) FOR OPIOID OVERDOSE

Narcan®, naloxone hydrochloride, administered intravenously in an initial dose of 0.4–0.8 mg rapidly reverses the neurologic and cardiorespiratory depression that can be fatal in an opioid overdose within about 2 minutes. Reversing the effects of the more potent opioids, such as fentanyl, or the longer acting, such as methadone, may take longer and call for a higher dose.

How it Works

Naloxone is a potent opioid antagonist. Essentially, its molecules will bind with the patients opioid receptor sites and literally kick out the opioid molecules out of the receptor sites and keep them out. If the opioid is a short-acting drug such as morphine or heroin, it will then remain in the bloodstream until it is metabolized and excreted. If the opioid is a longer-acting drug, such as methadone or LAAM, the drug may outlast the antagonist and the patient could then go back into overdose. Consequently, the overdose victim should be kept under observation at least until after the antagonist has worn off or at least 6 hours. Another reason for maintaining observation is the potential for triggering a significant withdrawal syndrome. Withdrawal and detoxification from opioids and other drugs will be the topic of Part II of this chapter.

The Role of Tolerance in Opioid Overdose

Habitual opioid users will develop tolerance to the drugs over time. As opioid tolerance develops, forcing the user to use increased quantities in order to achieve desired effects, the amount of drug that they can take in without compromise increases as well, so that if an overdose occurs it may involve relatively massive amounts of drug. Often an overdose in a habitual user results from the introduction of particularly pure drug that is much more potent than what the user is physiologically used to. Conversely, when an opioid addict undergoes detoxification and has remained drug free, the tolerance may drop rapidly, leaving the user vulnerable to overdose at drug amounts well below those taken during habitual use. Many overdoses occur during slips when users in relapse try to use at the level they maintained at the end of their habitual use.

■ SEDATIVE-HYPNOTIC INTOXICATION AND OVERDOSE

Keeping in mind that alcohol fits within the sedative-hypnotic family of drugs, the symptoms of intoxication and overdose are similar. For all, mild intoxication presents with slurred speech, ataxia, and incoordination. A state of paradoxical agitated confusion and possible delirium may occur, particularly in older patients. The symptoms may progress into overdose, characterized by stupor and coma, ultimately leading to potentially fatal respiratory arrest or cardiovascular collapse. As with opioids, the habitual user develops tolerance to the drug of choice and cross-tolerance to all other sedative-hypnotic drugs. Unlike the opioid tolerance, however, in sedative-hypnotic tolerance the amount of drug that the user can safely take does not increase along with the amount of drug needed to achieve desired effects. Consequently, over time and with habitual use, the amount of drug needed may approach a lethal level so that toxicity and overdose can occur with only small increases over regular intake.[6]

Synergistic Overdose

As with opioid overdose, sedative-hypnotic overdose is a potentially fatal occurrence. The benzodiazepines, currently a therapeutic workhorse because of their comparative safety, rarely cause death by themselves, but are often a major cause of fatal overdose because they act synergistically with other drugs, including alcohol, major tranquilizers, antidepressants, or opioids. In general, mixed overdoses among these various drugs are the most dangerous because combinations of these drugs allow one of the pair to build up into fatal concentrations in the brain while the liver is busy metabolizing the other.

Treating Intoxication and Overdose

Any sedative-hypnotic overdose is a life-threatening event and should be treated as such. Assessment, maintenance of airway and as necessary, ventilatory support should be the first consideration. The next step should be evacuation of the GI tract with a large-bore orogastric tube if a gag reflex is elicited or the airway is protected by intubation. A slurry of 1.0 g/kg activated charcoal together with a dose of cathartic should be given while repeated doses of activated charcoal, at 0.5–1.0 g/kg every 2–4 hours or by slow continuous nasogastric infusion, particularly for barbiturate or other non-benzodiazepine ingestions. Benzodiazepines can slow gut motility while phenobarbital, meprobamate, blutethimide, and ethchlorvynol can form concretions in the stomach. While alkalization of the urine may be helpful in eliminating phenobarbital, forced diureses has not been helpful in eliminating any sedative-hypnotics. Serum level measurement can be helpful in identifying and quantifying the ingested drug or drugs, but emergency clinical management should be based on the patient's condition, not on serum levels.[6]

Alcohol Overdose Management

With alcohol overdose there may be nausea and vomiting as well as ataxia. At potentially fatal serum levels, which may vary depending on the alcohol tolerance of the individual, progressive obtundation develops, accompanied by decreases in respiration, blood pressure and body temperature, urinary incontinence or retention and decreased or absent reflexes. Because of the depressed gas reflex the individual may vomit and aspirate the vomitus, thereby blocking the airway. Acute alcohol poisoning, particularly in binge drinkers, such as youth who "chug-a-lug" alcohol at a social gathering, can be fatal. The most important goal is preventing severe respiratory depression and protecting the airway against aspiration. Given the rapidity of alcohol absorption from the gut, emesis or gastric lavage is not usually indicated unless there has been major ingestion within the previous 30–60 minutes or the ingestion of other drugs is suspected. Use of stimulants ranging from amphetamine to the classic coffee may overcome some of the sedative or psychomotor impairment in acute alcohol intoxication, but is not clinically useful and may in fact result in a mixed CNS depressant/stimulant intoxication.[7]

Utilization of a Benzodiazepine Antagonist

Flumazenil has proved to be a competitive antagonist with weak agonist properties capable of reversing benzodiazepine sedative effects, however, it will have no effect on alcohol or other sedative-hypnotics. Its antagonist effects last only 30–60 minutes and its use has been associated with seizures and cardiac arrhythmias, so any use should be very carefully monitored, particularly with habitual benzodiazepine users, as they are at especially high risk for adverse effects.

■ ACUTE STIMULANT, HALLUCINOGEN, MARIJUANA, AND PHENCYCLIDINE EVENTS

You will notice that problems occurring during the direct use of these drugs are not referred to as overdoses. Diverse as they are, all of these drugs can produce acute events, and some of them may be fatal, but fatalities result from other factors than overdose. Following the designation used by Wilkins and colleagues in the *Principles of Addiction Medicine,* the authors will refer to these events and their treatment as management of stimulant, hallucinogen, marijuana, and phencyclidine intoxication.[8] In all cases, treatment for intoxication of these drugs should provide a means of medical intervention for initiating treatment for chronic use of these drugs.

Managing Stimulant Intoxication

Unlike opioids and sedative hypnotics, which are post-synaptic drugs, stimulants are pre-synaptic in their neuropharmacologic actions. Where the first two groups bind with receptor sites to produce their effects, stimulants have their effect at the pre-synaptic level by stimulating the release of the brain's own catecholamine neurotransmitter system. In other words, the stimulant effects are actually produced by the same neurotransmitters that are activated in fright, flight, and sexual arousal and activity. The effects are attenuated in cocaine use by a cocaine-mediated blockade of the neurotransmitter reuptake pumps. Once released, the stimulant neurotransmitters cannot return to their point of origin. Instead they continue to activate receptor sites until they are eaten by enzymes that clean up the spaces between brain cells, much like little pac-men roving through intersynaptic space.

Psychiatric and Behavioral Effects of Stimulant Intoxication

The effects of stimulant intoxication may be a combination of psychological and behavioral and physical. Psychiatric complications can range from behavioral disinhibition (an extension of the often desired disinhibition euphoria), bruxism, and hypervigilance to compulsive behavior, paranoia with delusions, ideas of reference and hallucinations, and stimulant psychosis (including dysfunction, hallucinosis, delusional behavior and either suicidal or homicidal responses). Stimulant psychosis can be mistaken for acute schizophrenia, but will subside with abstinence. Panic reactions, exacerbated by the physical symptoms of stimulant intoxication such as increased heartbeat and hyperventilation, can escalate into panic disorder.[9] The most common hallucinations are auditory or tactile, while visual hallucinations are rare and may suggest a possible neurologic etiology. Tactile hallucinations often take the form of insects crawling under the patient's skin.

Symptoms of severe intoxication can include a delirium syndrome similar to that found with phencyclidine (PCP) characterized by extreme emotional lability, enhanced strength, decreased awareness of pain and unpredictable, often violent behavior.[10] Schuckit[9] points out that high doses of either cocaine or amphetamines can precipitate an organic brain syndrome (OBS). Patients should be evaluated for intracranial bleeding and pre-existing neurological disease or psychopathology before initiating pharmacological treatment. According to Wilkins and colleagues,[8] "The OBS generally is self-limited, with treatment following the guidelines as for other OBS."

Physical Effects of Stimulant Intoxication

Acute stimulant intoxication may be accompanied by hyperthermia, vasoconstriction, hypertension, tachycardia, and heart palpitations. Of these, hyperthermia may occur independently and suggest a more severe prognosis, leading to reversible coagulopathy and renal failure. Other symptoms may include myocardial ischemia, arrhythmia, dyspnea, and in severe cases progress to cardiogenic shock, myocardia infarction, and death. Other systemic effects may include cerebral and pulmonary edema, hemorrhage, rhabdomyolysis, myoglobinuria, nephrotoxicity, and hyperkalemia.[11]

Treatment of Acute Stimulant Intoxication

Thus far, no antagonists have been developed to combat the presynaptic stimulants, making management of acute episodes that much more difficult. Once such possible medical problems as hyperthyroidism or pre-existing psychopathology have been ruled out and the presence of stimulants confirmed, the patient exhibiting symptoms of stimulant psychosis should be isolated within a calm, non-threatening atmosphere with sensory stimuli minimized. Treatment staff should be calm and confident but alert for possible aggressive outbursts. Physical restraints can increase the risk of hyperthermia and rhabdomyolysis and should be avoided unless absolutely necessary. Treatment itself should consist of reassurance that the effects will dissipate as the drug leaves the body. If reassurance proves inadequate, Shuckit[9] recommends anti-anxiety drug, such as chlordiazepoxide (10–25 mg orally) or diazepam (10–30 mg orally) be administered as needed every 30–60 minutes. As previously described, the Rock Medicine Section of the Haight Ashbury Free Clinics uses i.m. injection of 2 and 2 (2 mg Ativan and 2 mg Haldol). Neuroleptics should not be administered, as their use may exacerbate the sympathomimetic and cardiovascular effects of cocaine, producing hyperthermia and rapid death. The patient should be hospitalized and kept under observation until the episode of stimulant psychosis has passed. If the symptoms continue longer than 4–5 days following the last use of stimulants, the patient most likely has a non-drug-related problem.

Usually, the psychiatric symptoms constitute a first phase of intoxication with acute physical symptoms as the second and potentially more directly life-threatening phase. As we have seen, the medical effects of acute stimulant intoxication can be many, varied and life threatening. Responses are essentially of a symptom response basis, with the first priority being the maintenance of basic life-support functions, including airway patency and ventilation and close monitoring of vital signs, particularly cardiac and neurologic status, and treatment for shock if needed. Oral temperatures in excess of 102°F need to be aggressively managed through such means as external body cooling with ice packs or cold water, ice water gastric lavage, and hypothermic blankets. Diazepam i.v., 5–10 mg no more than 5 mg/min, can be used for seizures, as well as alternate therapies for repeated seizures, including intubation, or phenytoin or a short-acting barbiturate such as pentobarbital sodium (25–50 mg, i.v.). Hypertension lasting more than 15 minutes should be treated. Standard approaches are recommended for treating cocaine-associated myocardial ischemia, but use of beta-adrenergic blockers should be avoided. Treatment initially includes oxygen, benzodiazepine for sedation, nitroglycerin for vasodilation, and aspirin for anti-platelet action, during evaluation, followed by phentolamine and/or verapamil to reverse cocaine-induced coronary artery vasoconstriction. Angioplasty or thrombolysis can be performed if a diagnosis of myocardial infarction is established.

Obviously, the clinical picture can be confusing, patient history unreliable or impossible to obtain in an emergency situation. Urine and blood samples should always be obtained and toxicological analysis initiated as soon as possible.

Hallucinogen Acute Intoxication

Thankfully, in most cases the physical complications of hallucinogen acute intoxication are much less severe than those of stimulant drugs. Life-threatening overdoses on hallucinogens are rare, but they do happen, as do idiosyncratic allergic reactions to such drugs as MDMA.

The most common acute psychological and behavioral effects of hallucinogen intoxication are anxiety attacks or panic reactions in which the user feels out of control and in fear of permanent brain damage.

■ IMMEDIATE AND CHRONIC PROBLEMS WITH HALLUCINOGENS

In 1967, David E. Smith, M.D., identified the adverse effects of hallucinogens as "largely psychological in nature," and classified them as either acute toxicity, effects occurring during the use of the drug, or chronic after-effects.[12] Although there have been some occurrences of physiological consequences, particularly with MDMA, these have been primarily of an idiosyncratic nature, while in most cases the adverse effects of these drugs still appear to be psychological.

The acute toxic effects take many forms. Often individuals knowingly take a hallucinogenic drug and find themselves in a state of anxiety as the powerful hallucinogen begins to take effect. They were aware that they had taken a drug, but felt that they could not control its effects. This condition is similar to that of not being able to wake up from a threatening dream. Some users experiencing a bad trip try to physically flee the situation, giving rise to potential physical danger. Others may become paranoid and suspicious of their companions or other individuals.

Not all acute toxicity is based on anxiety or loss of control. Some people taking hallucinogens display decided changes in cognition and demonstrate poor judgment. They may decide that they can fly, and jump out of a window. Some users are reported to have walked into the sea, feeling that they were "at one of the universe." Such physical mishaps have been described within the acid culture as "being God, but tripping over the furniture." Susceptibility to bad trips is not necessarily dose related, but can depend on the experience, maturity, and personality of the user as well as "set and setting," i.e., the circumstances and the environment in which the trip takes place. Sometimes the individual will complain of unpleasant symptoms while intoxicated and later speak in glowing terms of the experience. Negative psychological set and environmental setting are the most significant contributing factors to bad hallucinogenic trips.[13]

■ TREATMENT OF ACUTE TOXICITY

Techniques originally developed within the psychedelic community and adopted by free clinics and other counter-culture-oriented treatment centers are based on the findings that most psychedelic bad trips are best treated in a supportive, non-pharmacological fashion through the restoration of a positive, non-threatening environment. Facilities, such as those occupied by the Haight Ashbury Free Clinics, in a residential setting with little to mark them as *medical*, with a quiet space or calm center set aside for drug crises and with casually dressed staff dedicated to a non-judgmental attitude were admirably suited for such treatment. At large rock concerts, emergency talkdown procedures are accomplished by Haight Ashbury staff and volunteers in a quiet space set up specifically for treating acute psychedelic toxicity. Talkdowns of most acute toxicity reactions can be accomplished without medication or hospitalization. Paraprofessionals with psychedelic drug experience have been particularly effective at such sites as large rock concerts. Amelioration of bad trips has even been accomplished by long-distance telephone calls.

In the talkdown approach, one should maintain a relaxed, conversational tone aimed at putting the individual at ease. Quick movements should be avoided. One should make the patient comfortable, but not impede their freedom of movement. Let them walk around, stand, sit or lie, down. At times, such physical movement and activity may be enough to break the anxiety reaction. Gentle suggestion should be used to divert patients from any activity that seems to be adding to their agitation. Getting the individual's mind off the frightening elements of a bad trip and onto positive elements is the key to the talkdown.

An understanding of the phases generally experienced in an hallucinogenic drug trip is most helpful in treating acute reactions. After orally ingesting an average dose of 100–250 μg of LSD, the user experiences sympathomimetic, or stimulant responses, including elevated heart rate and respiration. Adverse reactions in this phase are primarily managed by reassurances that these are normal and expected effects of psychedelic drugs. This reassurance is usually sufficient to override a potentially frightening situation.

From the first to the sixth hour, visual imagery becomes vivid and may take on frightening content. The patient may have forgotten taking the drug, and given acute time distortion, may believe this state will go on forever. Such fears can be dispelled by reminding the individual that these effects are drug induced, by suggesting alternative images and by distracting the individual from those images that are frightening.

In the later stages, philosophical insights and ideas predominate. Adverse experiences here are most frequently due to recurring unpleasant thoughts or feelings that can become overwhelming in their impact. The therapist can be most effective by being supportive and by suggesting new trains of thought.

The therapist's attitude toward hallucinogens and their use is very important. Empathy and self-confidence are essential. Anxiety and fear in the therapist will be perceived in an amplified manner by the client. Physical contact with the individual is often reassuring, but can be misinterpreted. Ideally, the therapist should rely on intuition rather than preconceptions.

Wesson and Smith[14] noted that medication may be necessary and should be given either after the talkdown has failed or as a supplement to the talkdown process. During the first phase of intervention, oral administration of a sedative, such as 25 mg of chlordiazepoxide (Librium®) or 10 mg of diazepam (Valium®), can have an important pharmacological and reassuring effect.

During the second and third phases, a toxic psychosis or major break with reality may occur in which one can no longer communicate with the individual. If the individual begins acting in such a way as to be an immediate danger, antipsychotic drugs may be employed. Only if the individual refuses oral medication and is out of behavioral control should anti-psychotics be administered by injection. Haloperidol (Haldol®) (2.0–4.0 mg administered intramuscularly every hour) is the current drug of choice. Any medication, however, should only be given by qualified personnel. If anti-psychotic drugs are required, hospitalization is usually indicated.

As soon as rapport and verbal contact are established, further medication is generally unnecessary. Occasionally, an individual fails to respond to the above regimen and must be referred to an inpatient psychiatric facility. Such a decision must be weighed carefully, however, as transfer to a hospital may of itself have an aggravating and threatening effect. Hospitalization should only be used as a last resort if all else has failed.

■ TREATING CHRONIC HALLUCINOGENIC DRUG AFTEREFFECTS

Chronic hallucinogenic drug aftereffects present situations wherein a condition that may be attributable to the ingestion of a toxic substance occurs or continues long after the metabolization of that substance. With the use of hallucinogens, five recognized chronic reactions have been reported: (1) prolonged psychotic reactions; (2) depression sufficiently severe so as to be life-threatening; (3) flashbacks; (4) exacerbations of pre-existing psychiatric illness; and (5) post-hallucinogen perceptual disorder.

Some people who have taken many hallucinogenic drug trips, especially those who have had acute toxic reactions, show what appears to be serious long-term personality disruptions. These prolonged psychotic reactions have similarities to schizophrenic reactions and appear to occur most often in people with pre-existing psychological difficulties, such as primarily pre-psychotic or psychotic personalities. Hallucinogenic drug-induced personality disorganizations can be quite severe and prolonged. Appropriate treatment often requires antipsychotic medication and residential care in a mental health facility followed by outpatient counseling.

At the Haight Ashbury Free Clinics, staff found that some of the clients self-medicated their hallucinogenic-precipitated psychotic episodes with amphetamines. Often this self-medication with amphetamines resulted in the development of amphetamine abuse, followed by secondary heroin, barbiturate, or alcohol abuse patterns to ameliorate the side effects of the amphetamines. Thus, in certain patients, chronic psychological problems induced by LSD and other hallucinogenic drugs can lead to complicated patterns of polydrug abuse that required additional treatment approaches.[15]

■ FLASHBACKS

By far the most ubiquitous chronic reaction to hallucinogens is the flashback. Flashbacks are transient spontaneous occurrences of some aspect of the hallucinogenic drug effect occurring after a period of normalcy that follows the original intoxication. This period of normalcy distinguishes flashbacks from prolonged psychotic reactions. Flashbacks may occur after a single ingestion of a psychedelic drug, but more commonly occur after multiple psychedelic drug ingestions.

Flashbacks are a symptom, not a specific disease entity. They may well have multiple causes, and many cases called flashbacks may have occurred although the individual had never ingested a psychedelic drug. Some investigators have suggested that flashbacks may be due to a residue of the drug, retained in the body and released into the brain at a later time. Although this is known to happen with phencyclidene (PCP) and drugs similar to it, there is no direct evidence of retention or prolonged storage of such psychedelics as LSD.

Individuals who have used psychedelic drugs several times a month have indicated that fleeting flashes of light and afterimage prolongation occurring in the periphery of vision commonly occur for days or weeks after ingestion. Active and chronic psychedelic drug users tend to accept these occurrences as part of the psychedelic experience, are unlikely to seek medical or psychiatric treatment and frequently view them as "free trips." It is the inexperienced user and the individual who attaches a negative interpretation to these visual phenomena who are likely to be disturbed by them and seek medical or psychiatric help. While emotional reactions to the flashback are generally contained with the period of the flashback itself, prolonged anxiety states or psychotic breaks have occurred following a frightening flashback. There is no record of flashback activity specifically attributable to hallucinogenic drug use occurring more than a year after the individual's last use of a psychedelic drug.[16]

■ LONG-TERM CONSEQUENCES OF HALLUCINOGENIC DRUG USE

The long-term study of adverse hallucinogenic drug reactions has revealed the existence of low prevalence, but quite disabling chronic consequences of LSD use. Of particular concern is the post-hallucinogen perceptual disorder (PHPD). With PHPD, individuals describe a persistent perceptual disorder which they describe as being like living in a bubble under water. They also describe trails of light and images following movement of their hands, and often describe living in a purple haze. This perceptual disorder is aggravated by any psychoactive drug use, including alcohol and marijuana, and is distinguished from flashbacks, which are episodic rather than chronic phenomena. With the PHPD, the individual often experiences anxiety, even panic, and becomes phobic and depressed. With the PHPD sufferers, our experience has been that individuals do not have a disturbed psychiatric history prior to the onset of psychedelic drug use and that the PHPD can occur even after a single dose.

With the more severe, prolonged LSD reactions, such as an LSD precipitated schizophrenic reaction, or severe depressive disorder, individuals almost always have a premorbid psychiatric history and require inpatient treatment. With the prolonged psychotic reactions, antipsychotic medication is required, and with the prolonged depressive reactions, antidepressant medication is required. A major concern involves teenagers with depressive reactions to psychedelic use that may result in severe depression culminating in suicide.

With the post-hallucinogen perceptual disorder, drug-free recovery with supportive counseling is often adequate treatment, although recovery may take several months and antianxiety medication may be needed to treat the secondary anxiety and panic disorder which develops when the individuals feel that they are irreversibly brain-damaged and will never see normally again.

■ TREATMENT ISSUES WITH MDMA

In that much recent hallucinogen use and therefore concomitant clinical research has focused on the psychological and psychiatric consequences of MDMA and related substances, the authors will devote some specific focus to that family of substances.

The first problem area is *Acute MDMA Toxicity*, which is essentially the result of taking too much MDMA in too short a period of time. This results in some physical or psychological dysfunction. The symptoms appear to be time/dose related. These symptoms range from a mild caffeine-like toxicity to potentially life-threatening stimulant overdoses.

The second area of concern is the *Prolonged MDMA Toxicity*, a result of chronic or regular ingestion of MDMA. The symptoms range in severity from mild dysphoria to frank paranoid psychosis and relate to both acute toxicity, chronicity of use and secondary drug effects such as sleep and appetite suppression.

The third problem area is the *MDMA-Induced Anxiety Syndromes*. These are problems related to MDMA's ability to bring unconscious material to consciousness. We have hypothesized that these anxiety syndromes are primarily caused by the lack of resolution and integration of now-conscious and often emotionally potent materials. These anxiety syndromes appear to be psychodynamic in nature and not purely toxicological. They last beyond the period of actual drug intoxication.[17]

■ LOW-DOSE ACUTE TOXICITY

Low-dose toxic reactions may include jitteriness, mild anxiety, mild apprehension, and jaw clenching. Because many MDMA users view the MDMA use as a relatively important event and many users even formally ritualize such use, an anticipation and apprehension of the events to come may blend with the sympathomimetic properties of MDMA to further heighten apprehension and perhaps even produce fear in predisposed people. Generally, most of the sympathomimetic reactions are dose-related, and are typically mild. Non-medicinal approaches, such as support, quiet and reassurance that the symptoms will fade over time, should be successful in reducing this apprehension. In most cases, individuals taking MDMA at the dosages that were previously used in therapy, i.e., 50–150 mg, would be aware that problems they may be experiencing are drug-related.

■ MEDIUM-DOSE ACUTE TOXICITY

At somewhat higher doses, i.e., 250–300 mg. MDMA, dose and setting-related psychopathology may develop. In a person with low tolerance to stimulants, there may be a Medium-Dose Acute Toxicity resulting from ingestion at this level.

Visual distortions have been reported, such as viewing an object that appears to be shimmering, shiny or perhaps moving in a jittery fashion, or with geometric embellishments. There is an awareness that these distortions are drug-induced, and they do not appear to carry any particularly positive or negative content. Also, they do not typically interfere with the therapeutic goals of insight and empathy for most individuals. Some users have reported that they desire to be alone and some report that they become slightly concerned about others noticing their behavior and knowing that they are "high." There can be a slightly paranoid flavor or self-conscious tendency which appears to be dose-related. These feelings of self-consciousness may only occur while inside a building or in crowds, and there may be a tendency to move outdoors.

For many, there may be a fairly distressing depression which may emerge rapidly, especially if there is a sudden shift in con-sciousness away from the particularly empathic or euphoric stage of the MDMA experience. The subjective aspect of this depression may have to do with returning to a fairly normal con-sciousness after having experienced often significantly beautiful and/or meaningful feelings.

■ **HIGH-DOSE ACUTE TOXICITY**

The most obvious and most clinically important acute toxicolo-gical problem involves the high-dose MDMA toxic reaction. Depending upon personal variables such as prior drug experi-ence (especially with stimulants, hallucinogens and PCP), toler-ance to the effects of the drug and setting, the toxic range for MDMA may be as low as 300 mg for some people, but 400 mg or more for others. Toxic symptomatology would be on a conti-nuum ranging from anxiety symptoms and panic with or without tachycardia to psychotic reactions with paranoia and violence. Hypertensive crises and even cerebrovascular accidents and cardiac arrhythmia could theoretically occur as with cocaine and the amphetamines.

Some MDMA users may also use other drugs during the same time period. Others may use MDMA in combination with other drugs, such as MDA or marijuana. Other drugs that may have similar properties and effects to those of MDMA include 2-CB, or 4-bromo-2,5-dimethoxyphenethylamine and MDE (Eve) or N-ethyl-3,4-methylenedioxy-methamphetamine.

■ TREATMENT CONSIDERATIONS

The medical management of this problem will also be on a continuum. At the lower doses or at the least severe reactions, the appropriate medical management of the client may simply be a supportive, reassuring interaction with the subject, moving him/her to a perceived safe environment and reducing stimuli. The person should be told that the distressing symptoms will fade over time. It would be optimal if someone with psychotherapeutic skills were to spend time with the subject, given that potent psychodynamic issues may come forth. It would be best if the person is not left alone, but with someone who is capable of providing psychological support.

For moderately dysfunctional anxiety symptoms which increase with severity, 5–10 mg diazepam may be given orally. For the patient who also experiences tachycardia, propanalol, 10–20 mg, can be given orally, or if given i.v., administer from 0.5–1 mg very slowly at a maximum of 1 mg per minute up to a total of 6 mg.

If the symptoms are more severe, consideration should be given to containment if (1) anxiety merges into aggressive behavior, (2) evidence of stimulant psychosis with violence to self or to others, and (3) there are suicidal verbalizations or behaviors. If the client has a *stimulant psychosis,* and is markedly anxious, either: (A) Give haloperidol 2 mg b.i.d. and 2 mg i.m. of a short-acting benzodiazepine like Ativan or 5-10 mg i.v. of a longer-acting benzodiazepine like diazepam, and assess remaining anxiety, treating with diazepam 5–10 mg i.v. if necessary or (B) give

5–10 mg diazepam orally or i.v. If anxiety is still marked, give diazepam every 1–2 hours. If anxiety is effectively treated, give diazepam every 4–6 hours for a maximum of about 40 mg per 24 hour period. If stimulant psychosis remains and is an issue relative to violence or danger to self or others, give haloperidol 2 mg b.i.d. orally.

For persistent adrenergic crisis, give propanalol orally in doses of 40–60 mg at 4–6 hour intervals for duration of crisis. A pulse of 90 or less is the goal. Many stimulant psychosis patients will be resistant to haloperidol and may in fact request a seda-tive-hypnotic to reduce anxiety. Some of these patients may be able to handle the stimulant psychosis if anxiolytic therapy is given. The important diagnosis criterion is: Does the psychotic break represent a clear danger to the client or to others? Also note that the amphetamines and haloperidol both lower seizure threshold, so caution should be used. Also, some patients may be very sensitive to the sedative-hypnotics and proceed into coma with even lower doses than recommended, thus caution is urged.

■ PROLONGED HIGH-DOSE MDMA TOXICITY

The person who uses high doses of MDMA (or any mood-altering drug) on a daily basis is a person likely to have a substance abuse disorder. Whereas most people who use MDMA for its psychother-apeutic benefits dislike the stimulant properties of MDMA, some people actively seek out this experience. Clearly, present cocaine problems speak to the fact that stimulant abuse is commonplace. In interviews with MDMA users, it was revealed that some cocaine dealers also sold MDMA as an adjunct to their normal trade, and many cocaine abusers and addicts were introduced to MDMA in this setting. Also, amphetamine addicts who have had access to MDMA may have used MDMA as an alternative to amphetamine or turned to MDMA as a supplement to their amphetamine use. Because drug switching is a regular part of drug abuse, a regular stimulant abuser might have a tendency to use MDMA at higher doses and for longer periods of time, and to use this drug for its stimulant rather than its empathogenic qualities. These individuals might also exhibit a cross-tolerance to MDMA and thus be able to ingest fairly large quantities of the drug.

The daily or chronic use of a CNS stimulant can push a person to the limit and drain their physical and psychological strengths. With the high-dose chronic user, mood swings, emotional lability, and anxiety can increase, trading off with the depression in times of abstinence. In time, stimulant psychosis, paranoia, and violence could emerge.

■ PROLONGED LOW-DOSE MDMA TOXICITY

While high-dose chronic use of MDMA suggests stimulant addiction, the lower dose extended use may suggest a different type of drug use. The stimulant addict understands and desires the stimulant effects of amphetamines and cocaine. That is not the case with a number of people we have interviewed. Most often, these are individuals engaged in generalized drug experimentation and their chronic use is usually over a finite period of time, usually a week or two.

The effects of this prolonged MDMA use at lower doses include mild psychopathology. Interviewees describe a lack of mental clarity, being "out of sorts," having mild mental confusion and slight memory impairment. Some mention a lack of motivation, mild disorientation, and forgetfulness. There may be some sleep dysfunction and some nutritional needs may not be met if the pattern continues. They did not report anxiety or hyperactivity, however, and that may be due to titrating or controlling their doses over the day. They also state that cessation of MDMA use returns them to their normal emotions and psychological state.

■ TREATMENT CONSIDERATIONS

It is important that the possible presence of addictive disease be assessed. The chronicity of use, as opposed to event-specific use or very rare use, may be a signal of addictive illness. Appropriate treatment for the addiction would include inpatient or outpatient chemical dependency treatment based on an abstinence model of supported recovery. Appropriate referral should be made to such 12-Step programs as Alcoholics Anonymous or Narcotics Anonymous.

MDMA-Induced Anxiety Syndromes

For some users, MDMA will bring to the surface unconscious material that may manifest itself in a variety of negative ways. These problems seem unrelated to volume, dose, or duration of MDMA use. We have identified it as a delayed anxiety disorder secondary to MDMA ingestion. In these cases, the MDMA user reports one or more symptoms of anxiety, typically emerging shortly after their initial MDMA experience. These symptoms range from a mild anxiety or concentration difficulties to a full-blown disorder such as panic attack with hyperventilation and tachycardia, phobic disorders, parasthesias, or other anxiety states. In one case, reported by therapist Lincoln Beals to Richard Seymour, the subject self-medicated the MDMA reactions with increasing amounts of MDMA, coupled with other psychoactive drugs, and eventually died of "terminal insight."

In some cases, the client will be particularly concerned about a certain part of the body. The client may perceive that a hand is shaking, or that the extremities are cold and clammy. Subjective reactions to these concerns can range from mildly annoying to highly inhibiting. The dysfunction may require psychiatric or psychological intervention.

Medical Effects of Hallucinogens

Acute medical complications to LSD are rare but convulsions and hyperthermia (characterized by dry skin, increased muscle tone, agitation, and seizures) do occur. Body temperature should be monitored. Given the low (microgram level) dosages and rapid absorption with LSD, gastric lavage and ipecac-induced vomiting are not indicated. MDMA-related medical emergencies usually involve hyperthermia, seizures, cardiac arrhythmia, disseminated intravascular coagulation, rhabdomyolysis, and acute renal failure. MDMA emergencies can be fatal. Given the high potential for dehydration in connection with hyperthermia resulting from prolonged exertion at "raves," patients with possible MDMA toxicity should receive intravenous fluids and dantrolene, and if necessary treated with tepid wet towels, ice packs, cooling sponge baths, and rectal acetaminophen.[18]

■ MARIJUANA ACUTE INTOXICATION

Oral ingestion may cause more acute effects than smoking. However, psychotic states as a result of marijuana use are rare. Most adverse reactions consist of depersonalization, acute panic and anxiety, and in large or particularly potent doses, delirium. Time and space distortion, visual and auditory hallucinations, and some paranoia are all possible. There are no recognized cases of cannabis overdose fatality and the physiological effects of acute intoxication are usually mild. Possibly because of the lack of acute problems, marijuana use often becomes chronic and destructive in the long term.

■ TREATMENT OF ACUTE MARIJUANA INTOXICATION

Currently the best treatment for acute marijuana problems is similar to that for hallucinogens, i.e., supportive reassurance. A highly specific cannabinoid receptor antagonist that blocks the acute effects of marijuana in animals in much the way naloxone works in an opioid overdose (SR141716A) is presently undergoing initial Phase I human trials. If this or another compound proves to be safe and effective, it could be used to treat extreme cases of marijuana intoxication.

■ PHENCYCLIDINE (PCP) INTOXICATION

Phencyclidine and its cogeners, including ketamine, which has similar effects, are very complex drugs, acting at varying dosages or varying amounts in the body as a stimulant, a sedative and a hallucinogen. Unlike the hallucinogens, such as LSD, mescaline and psilocybin, and the hallucinogenic stimulants, such as MDA, etc.,

PCP acts as a mind/body dissociative. The hallucinating user may have no grounding, no sense of having taken a drug and no clear sense that his or her hallucinations are unreal.

Intoxication has been observed to occur in three stages: (1) conscious, with psychological effects but mild physiological effects; (2) stuporous or in a light coma, but responsive to pain; and (3) comatose and unresponsive to pain. Stage 1 intoxication may include nystagmus, hypertension, tachycardia, ataxia, dysarthria, numbness and hyperreflexia. The tachycardia and hypertension can be treated with beta-blockers or calcium channel blockers. In general, Stage 1 should be treated non-pharmacologically with reassuring, reality-oriented communication so long as the patient is receptive, in quiet isolation from external stimuli. Stages 2 and 3 are medical emergencies requiring comprehensive treatment in a medical setting that focuses on maintaining life-support functions and hastening the elimination of the PCP in the body. The latter can be accomplished by acidifying the patient's urine below pH 5 and utilizing forced diuresis by administering ammonium chloride (2.75 mEq/kg in 60 ml of saline every 6 hours through nasogastric tube and 2 g of i.v. ascorbic acid in 500 ml of IV fluid every 6 hours).[19] As a fat-soluble drug, PCP can stay in the body for long periods of time, so elimination becomes a key factor in both acute intoxication and chronic abuse.

■ DETOXIFICATION STRATEGIES

Incidents of acute intoxication are often a strong indication of chronic abuse. Whenever possible, the patient should be screened for drug use history and when appropriate urged to enter treatment. Generally, the first step in treating chronic abuse is detoxification. This means eliminating the drug from the body and mediating the symptoms of withdrawal, i.e., mediating the inevitable adjustments that the body must make in order to reestablish its balance once the drug is removed.

Most withdrawal symptoms are the opposite of the drug's desired effects. Imagine a pendulum that has been pulled way out of center. When that pendulum is released, it will swing a compensatory distance in the other direction before reaching equilibrium. Basically that is what happens in withdrawal, the body compensates by overreacting to every nuance that was suppressed by the drug. Physical detoxification is only part of early treatment. There is also dealing with mental withdrawal, but that will be discussed in the third section of this chapter.

For a long time, it was believed that only opioids and sedative-hypnotic drugs (including alcohol) produced withdrawal symptomatology. Today it is clear that all psychoactive drugs abused on a chronic basis will produce withdrawal syndromes. In the following section, the authors will discuss those syndromes and some basic withdrawal treatment protocols.

Opioid Withdrawal

The good news is that opioid withdrawal is not life-threatening. It can be accomplished either on an inpatient or outpatient basis. With short-term chronic use patients it can be accomplished within a non-medical treatment setting.

Craving is a key component in withdrawal, and the severity of withdrawal symptoms has a direct effect on the intensity of craving. In general, the withdrawal symptoms are the opposite of the opioid effects. They can include restlessness, irritability, insomnia, marked pupillary dilation, rhinorrhea, cutaneous and mucocutaneous lacrimation and piloerection, yawning, sneezing, nausea, vomiting, and diarrhea.

The duration of withdrawal depends on the drug of use. Meperidine abstinence syndrome may peak within 8–12 hours and continue for 4–5 days, while heroin symptoms peak at about 36–74 hours and may last 7–14 days. According to Schuckit[9] and a variety of others, there may be a protracted abstinence syndrome characterized by mild abnormalities in vital signs and continued craving, but this has not been clearly defined.

Treatment of opioid withdrawal ranges from a nonmedical, social model through symptomatic medication to methadone and LAAM maintenance. The decision of what protocol to follow depends on a number of factors, and calls for a thorough assessment of health and environmental conditions, including the presence of comorbid medical and psychiatric problems, availability of social support (such as presence of responsible family members who can provide monitoring and transportation) and polydrug abuse. Supportive measures include providing a safe environment and adequate nutrition, and a program of reassuring, supportive and effective treatment.

Medical Intervention

Starting at the far end, there are some cases in which detoxification does not seem to work, at least for the time being. The strategy in such cases is to defray withdrawal by shifting the patient from his or her drug of choice onto a long-acting opioid agonist, such as methadone or LAAM, that can be clinically administered and controlled. These agonists will at least provide some stability to the patient's life, by providing a means of avoiding withdrawal and decreasing craving and by occupying the opioid receptor sites so that use of illicit or other opioids will have no further effect. The patient can be maintained on methadone or LAAM until such time as detoxification becomes a feasible option.

Next in line is methadone detoxification. Here, methadone is substituted for the opioid of choice and then withdrawn over time. Withdrawal is managed with initial doses of 15–20 mg of methadone per day to control withdrawal symptoms for 2 or 3 days, then reduced by 10–15% per day, adjusted on the basis of symptom control and clinical findings. These are averages. Actual amounts and percentages depend on the amount of drug the patient has been using.

Clonidine, an alpha-2 agonist originally used in the treatment of hypertension is now used extensively in managing opioid withdrawal. Clonidine not only decreases withdrawal symptoms, it also seems to alleviate opioid craving. Usually administered for 10–14 days, and at a variety of dosages ranging from 0.2 mg orally every 4 hours up to a total daily dose of 1.2 mg, clonidine can then be tapered at a rate of approximately 0.2 mg per day depending on symptoms. One needs to watch for hypotension during administration. A benzodiazepine such as oxazepam may be helpful for insomnia and muscle cramps.

Clonidine is also used in combination with the long-acting opioid antagonist naltrexone in a form of rapid detoxification, developed to shorten the period of acute withdrawal to a period of around 5 days.

Several forms of "ultra-rapid detoxification" (URD) have been developed. In URD, the patient is placed under heavy sedation or general anesthesia, then given oral naltrexone or IV naloxone. The patient experiences acute withdrawal while in a sedated or unconscious state. It has been argued that such protocols do not allow a window of opportunity to treat psychological withdrawal during the course of detoxification, increasing the potential for relapse into active opioid addiction.

A new and very promising course of detoxification employs buprenorphine, a partial agonist with qualities similar to both methadone and naltrexone. Buprenorphine can be given once a day to block withdrawal symptoms and can act as a transitional agent between opioids and naltrexone.

Varieties and combinations of these detoxification protocols include symptomatic medication in differing combinations. At the Haight Ashbury Free Clinics, non-narcotic symptomatic medication using sedative and antispasmodic medicines is used in tandem with clonidine in one of several outpatient opioid detoxification protocols.

It should be kept in mind that physical detoxification is only part of the first step in treatment. The period of detoxification provides a window of opportunity to initiate the shift from active addiction to active recovery and should never be seen as an end in itself. The goal is to blend detoxification into ongoing drug treatment.

Sedative-Hypnotic Detoxification

The bad news is that sedative-hypnotic withdrawal, including that from alcohol addiction, can be life threatening. Sedative-hypnotic withdrawal symptoms are generally divided into major and minor categories. Minor withdrawal symptoms consist of anxiety, insomnia, tremor, and nightmares. A major withdrawal syndrome includes all the symptoms of minor withdrawal and may also include grand mal seizures, psychosis, hyperpyrexia, and death.

Untreated, the high-dose sedative-hypnotic withdrawal syndrome peaks in intensity as blood levels of the sedative drop, and the patient's signs and symptoms subside over a few days.

Symptoms attributed to sedative-hypnotic withdrawal include anxiety, tension, agitation, restlessness, irritability, tremor, nausea, insomnia, panic attacks, impairment of memory and concentration, perceptual alterations including hyperaculsis or hypersensitivity to touch and pain, paresthesias, feelings of unreality, visual hallucinations, psychosis, tachycardia, and increased blood pressure. Unfortunately, withdrawal has no pathognomonic signs or symptoms, and such a broad range of nonspecific symptoms could be produced by a number of illnesses, including agitated depression, generalized anxiety disorder, panic disorder, partial complex seizures, and schizophrenic disorders.

■ PATIENT EVALUATION

In that many individuals develop a sedative-hypnotic addiction at least in part iatrogenically, having been prescribed drugs in this category, it is particularly important to sort out the nuances of use and abuse. Eickelberg and Mayo-Smith[6] suggest the following steps for the evaluation and assessment of patients suspected of sedative-hypnotic addiction:

Step 1: Determine the reason(s) that the patient or referral source is seeking evaluation of sedative hypnotic use and/or discontinuation. Determine the indication(s) for the patient's drug use. A discussion with the referring physician should be standard practice. Discussion with any other referring person(s) or close family members often is helpful. Seek evidence to answer the question of whether the patient's use is improving the quality of his or her life or causing significant disability and/or exacerbating the original condition.

Step 2: Take a sedative-hypnotic use history, including, at a minimum, the dose, duration of use, substance(s) used and the patient's clinical response to sedative-hypnotic use currently and over time. The history should include any attempts at abstinence, symptoms experienced with changing the dose, and reasons for increasing or decreasing the dose. The history also should include behavioral responses to sedative-hypnotic use and any adverse or toxic side effects. For long-term users, a determination of the current pharmacological and clinical efficacy should be sought.

Step 3: Elicit a detailed accounting of other psychoactive drug use (including medical and non-medical, prescribed and over-the-counter drugs), as well as current use of alcohol and prior sequelae of use. The history also should include abstinence attempts and/or prior periods of abstinence, in addition to prior withdrawal experiences.

Step 4: Take a psychiatric history, including current and past psychiatric diagnoses, hospitalizations, suicide attempts, treatments, psychotherapy, and therapists (names and locations).

Step 5: Take a family history of substance use, psychiatric, and medical disorders.

Step 6: Take a current and past medical history of the patient, including illnesses, trauma, surgery, medications, allergies, and history of loss of consciousness, seizure(s), or seizure disorder.

Step 7: Take a psychosocial history, including current social status and support system.

Step 8: Perform a physical and mental status examination.

Step 9: Conduct a laboratory urine drug screen for substances of abuse. An alcohol Breathalyzer (if available) often is helpful in providing evidence of substance use which was not provided in the history. Depending on the patient's profile, EKG, HIV testing, TB testing, a blood chemistry panel, liver enzymes, CBC, and/or pregnancy testing may be indicated.

Step 10: Complete an individualized assessment, taking into account all aspects of the patient's presentation and history and, in particular, focusing on factors that would significantly influence the presence, severity, and time course of withdrawal.

Step 11: Arrive at a differential diagnosis, including a comprehensive listing of considered and/or possible diagnoses. This greatly aids and guides clinical management decisions as the patient's symptoms diminish, emerge or change in character during and after drug cessation.

Step 12: Determine the appropriate setting for detoxification.

Step 13: Determine the most efficacious detoxification method. In addition to proven clinical and pharmacological efficacy, the method selected should be one that the physician and clinical staff in the detoxification setting are comfortable with and experienced in administering.

Step 14: Obtain the patient's informed consent.

Step 15: Initiate detoxification. Ongoing physician involvement is central to appropriate management of detoxification. Subsequent to the patient assessment, development of the treatment plan, and obtaining patient consent, the individualized discontinuation program should be initiated. the physician closely monitors and flexibly manages (adjusting as necessary) the dosing or detoxification strategy to provide the safest, most comfortable and efficacious course of detoxification. To achieve optimal results, the physician and patient will need to establish a close working relationship.

The validity of a low-dose withdrawal syndrome has been controversial. Many people who have taken benzodiazepines in therapeutic doses for months to years can abruptly discontinue the drug without developing symptoms. Others, taking similar amounts of a benzodiazepine, develop a physical dependence on the drug and cannot tolerate the symptoms that develop when the drug is stopped or the dosage reduced. Moreover, some physicians believe the symptoms that emerge during the immediate withdrawal period can be explained solely by the return of the symptoms for which the drug was being taken, while other physicians propose that at least some of the symptoms are a true withdrawal reaction. At least four possible etiologies could explain the symptoms that begin when benzodiazepines are stopped. These are: symptom reemergence, symptom emergence, symptom overinterpretation, and symptom generation.

■ SYMPTOM REEMERGENCE

According to the symptom reemergence etiology, the patient's symptoms of anxiety, insomnia, or muscle tension abate during benzodiazepine treatment, and the patient forgets how severe they were. Because discomfort in the present seems more real than that experienced in the past, present symptoms may be perceived as more severe when, in fact, they are equal in severity to those experienced before treatment.

■ SYMPTOM EMERGENCE

If the patient's initial symptoms were secondary to a progressive disease, they may have been masked during benzodiazepine therapy. If this is the case, the symptoms that reemerge will be more intense when the drug is stopped, but the intensity will result from the disease's progression.

■ SYMPTOM OVERINTERPRETATION

Most individuals experience occasional anxiety, variations in sleep pattern, and musculoskeletal discomfort and accept these symptoms as reasonable consequences of every-day stresses, overexertion, or minor viral infections. Patients who are stopping sedative drugs often expect withdrawal symptoms to develop, and may assume that any symptoms occurring during the withdrawal period are caused by drug withdrawal and require medical attention. A study of the frequency with which symptoms attributed to minor barbiturate or low-dose benzodiazepine withdrawal actually occurred reported that many of the same nonspecific symptoms were common among untreated, healthy persons who did not use drugs.

■ SYMPTOM GENERATION

According to the final possible etiology, signs or symptoms may develop as a result of receptor site alterations caused by exposure to sedative-hypnotic drugs.

■ RECEPTOR-SITE MEDIATION IN DEPENDENCE AND WITHDRAWAL

Assigning causality to symptoms that emerge after discontinuing a drug is subject to uncertainty, especially when a patient is evaluated after dependence is already established. The time course of symptom resolution is the primary differentiating feature between symptoms generated by withdrawal and symptom reemergence, emergence or overinterpretation. Withdrawal symptoms subside with continued abstinence, whereas symptoms associated with other etiologies persist.

Such short-acting benzodiazepines as oxazepam, alprazolam, and triazolam have an accelerated time course for the sedative-hypnotic type of withdrawal syndrome, and the peak intensity of withdrawal occurs within 2–4 days. The fluctuation of symptom intensity of the low-dose withdrawal syndrome illustrates the waxing and waning of symptoms that often occurs without apparent psychological cause. This waxing and waning is an important marker distinguishing low-dose withdrawal symptoms from symptom reemergence.

Chronic use, dosage, concurrent drug use, and individual susceptibility all interact in the development of low-dose physical dependence. Moreover, the short-acting benzodiazepines are no less likely to produce physical dependence if taken on a daily basis than are the long-acting benzodiazepines, and once pharmacological dependence develops, the sedative-hypnotic-type withdrawal syndrome produced by short-acting benzodiazepines would be expected to be more intense because of the more rapid drop in tissue levels of these drugs.

■ BENZODIAZEPINE RECEPTOR SITES

Since the reports of finding specific benzodiazepine-binding sites the character of the benzodiazepine receptor site has been the subject of intense research. These receptor sites, localized in synaptic contact regions in the cerebral cortex, cerebellum, and hippocampus, are associated with gamma-aminobutyric acid (GABA) receptor sites and affect their affinity for binding to a specific site, and also modify the cell membrane's permeability to chloride ions. The authors have hypothesized that low-dose benzodiazepine withdrawal is receptor-site mediated. A receptor-site-mediated withdrawal syndrome could plausibly explain why benzodiazepine withdrawal symptoms take more time to resolve than non-benzodiazepine sedative-hypnotic withdrawal symptoms.

■ LOW-DOSE BENZODIAZEPINE DEPENDENCE SYNDROME

The low-dose benzodiazepine dependence syndrome is not well understood or well characterized. The dose–response relationship is not established, and the development of dependence appears to be idiosyncratic. Risk factors include a family or personal history of alcoholism, daily alcohol use, or concomitant use of other sedatives.

Because the time course and spectrum of signs and symptoms of the low-dose withdrawal syndrome are different from those of the sedative-hypnotic-type withdrawal syndrome, the two probably have different mechanisms. Thus, the low-dose benzodiazepine withdrawal syndrome should not be considered a "minor" sedative-hypnotic withdrawal syndrome, but a different syndrome. The benzodiazepine syndrome is not completely suppressed by phenobarbital administration; symptoms are rapidly reversed by benzodiazepine doses below those that would be expected to be effective; symptom resolution takes much longer with the low-dose withdrawal syndrome than with typical sedative-hypnotic withdrawal, i.e., symptoms usually take 6 months to a year to completely subside; and symptoms are most intense during withdrawal of the last few milligrams of the benzodiazepine.

■ BENZODIAZEPINE DETOXIFICATION

There are three accepted protocols for benzodiazepine detoxification. These are reduction of the amount of benzodiazepine taken, substitution of a longer-acting benzodiazepine, or substitution of phenobarbital. Some clinicians have also used carbamazine (an anticonvulsant) for prolonged withdrawal. Protocol selection depends on the severity of the benzodiazepine dependence, the involvement of other drugs of dependence, and the clinical setting in which the detoxification program takes place.

Given these variables, benzodiazepine withdrawal is no more controversial than alcohol withdrawal. As with alcohol detoxification, a minority of benzodiazepine users experience medically significant withdrawal. In that detoxification for that minority in both cases may involve life-threatening seizures, care must be taken in all withdrawal situations, and when needed, vital signs monitored during threshold periods of inpatient detoxification.

When a patient develops benzodiazepine dependence during treatment of anxiety, the physician must decide whether the patient should undergo detoxification. Abrupt cessation of long-term benzodiazepine use can produce severe and even life-threatening withdrawal sequelae.

The graded reduction of benzodiazepine protocol is used primarily in medical settings for therapeutic-dose dependence. Substituting a long-acting benzodiazepine (such as chlordiazepoxide) can be used to detoxify patients with primary benzodiazepine dependence, but is mainly used to treat patients with alcohol/benzodiazepine combination dependencies, using a fixed-dosage reduction schedule. Substitution of phenobarbital or another long-acting sedative-hypnotic can also be used to detoxify patients with primary benzodiazepine/polydrug dependence, for example, cocaine/benzodiazepine/alcohol combinations. This protocol, which also follows a fixed-dosage detoxification schedule, has the broadest use for all sedative-hypnotic drug dependencies and is widely used in drug detoxification programs. It is particularly valuable for treating high-dose benzodiazepine dependence.

If the theory about two benzodiazepine withdrawal syndromes, i.e., high-dose dependence of the barbiturate type and low-dose dependence, is correct, drug withdrawal strategies must be tailored to three possible dependence situations. After daily use of therapeutic doses of benzodiazepines for more than 6 months, only a low-dose withdrawal syndrome should be expected. After high-dose use, i.e., doses greater than the recommended therapeutic doses, for more than 1 month but less than 6 months, or for an average of 3 months, a classic sedative-hypnotic withdrawal syndrome should be anticipated. Finally, after daily high doses for more than 6 months, both a sedative-hypnotic withdrawal syndrome and a low-dose withdrawal syndrome should be anticipated.

To treat a low-dose dependence benzodiazepine withdrawal syndrome, gradual reduction of the benzodiazepine is pharmacologically rational because seizures, hyperpyrexia, and other life-threatening medical complications are not expected. A stepwise reduction of the drug by the smallest unit dose each week is recommended for patients who are pharmacologically dependent but still in control of their medication use. Patients who have lost the ability to control drug use are likely to escalate the dosage again as symptoms emerge, and they require hospitalization.

During withdrawal, psychometric assessment is useful for establishing trends in the multiple, shifting symptoms. A computer can be used to administer a symptom checklist, with the patient sitting at a terminal and entering responses. This interactive method has proved to be more efficient than interviews for tracking symptom changes.

Propanolol has been found to reduce symptom intensity,[20] and the drug is begun at a dosage of 20 mg every 6 hours, starting on the fifth day of withdrawal. This schedule is continued for 2 weeks and then stopped. After withdrawal is completed, propranolol is used as needed to control tachycardia, increased blood pressure, and anxiety. Continuous propranolol therapy for more than 2 weeks is not recommended, as propranolol itself may result in symptom rebound when discontinued after prolonged therapy.

Sedative-Hypnotic Detoxification with a Phenobarbital Taper

To treat sedative-hypnotic withdrawal, a phenobarbital substitution technique is preferred by the authors. At the Haight Ashbury Free Clinics, no patients have had withdrawal seizures when phenobarbital was used, whereas two patients have had seizures during gradual benzodiazepine reduction. When treating a patient for drug dependence, it is best not to administer the drug of dependence during treatment.

An estimate of the patient's daily benzodiazepine use during the month before treatment is used to compute the detoxification starting dose of phenobarbital, converting the benzodiazepine amount to the phenobarbital withdrawal equivalence dosage. The computed phenobarbital equivalence dosage is given in 3–4 doses daily. If other sedative-hypnotic drugs, including alcohol, are used, the amount of phenobarbital computed according to the conversion rate for the other sedative-hypnotic is added to the amount computed for the benzodiazepine. Regardless of the total computed amount, however, the maximum phenobarbital dosage is 500 mg per day. After 2 days of phenobarbital stabilization, the patient's daily dosage is decreased by 30 mg each day.

Before receiving each dose of phenobarbital, the patient is checked for sustained horizontal nystagmus, slurred speech, and ataxia. If sustained nystagmus is present, the scheduled dose of phenobarbital is withheld. If all three signs are present, the next two doses of phenobarbital are withheld and the daily dosage of phenobarbital for the following day is halved.[21]

Stimulant Withdrawal

Stimulant withdrawal may be characterized by a variety of non-specific aches and pains, tremors, chills, and involuntary motor movements, none of which should require specific medical treatment. Myocardial ischemia, with coronary vasospasm as a possible contributing factor, may occur during the first week of withdrawal. In general, the stimulant withdrawal syndrome results from the depletion of neurotransmitters, especially dopamine and may be treated with the dopamine agonists bromocriptine and amantadine. The best treatment regimen is supportive treatment and allowing the patient to sleep and eat as needed. Severe depression may occur and can be treated with antidepressants. Anhedonia, the inability to feel pleasure, may also appear. During the later stages of withdrawal, as the exhausted neurotransmitters are replenished, intense craving may occur, particularly in cocaine addicts, and these patients may need to be hospitalized in order to keep them from relapse. The time of withdrawal is, again, a window of opportunity to work on avoiding using cues and developing a sense of long-term abstinence and sobriety.

Withdrawal from Marijuana

Marijuana withdrawal is characterized by irritability, restlessness, anorexia, insomnia, diaphoresis, nausea, diarrhea, muscle twitches and flu-like symptoms, mild increases in heart rate, blood pressure, and body temperature. If a syndrome does develop, it usually manifests within 24 hours of cessation, peaks within 2–4 days and is over within 1–2 weeks. In general, the withdrawal is considered mild and rarely requires medical treatment or hospitalization. The greatest danger is relapse into severe psychological dependence. If severe insomnia develops, the serotonergic anti-depressant trazodone has been helpful.

Hallucinogens

Use of such hallucinogens as LSD tends to be intermittent. This may be due to the very rapid development of tolerance to these drugs precluding sufficiently chronic use as to form the basis of a withdrawal syndrome when use is discontinued. Consequently, there is no role for medication in treating hallucinogen withdrawal. Treatment can proceed directly to behavioral therapies.

Phencyclidine Withdrawal

The main thing to remember with phencyclidine withdrawal is that the drug remains in the body for a long time. In the early years of experience with PCP, the drug was thought to cause permanent brain damage. That assumption was only corrected as extreme cases "came back" over time. As was seen with hallucinogens, PCP experience can trigger long-lasting psychiatric sequelae, ranging from prolonged states of anxiety or depression to mild to pronounced psychotic states. These states can be dealt in psychosocial treatment, medicated only in extreme cases. Treatment of prolonged psychosis essentially follows guidelines for treating chronic functional psychosis. Flashback phenomena may be experienced up to a year after last use, but the effects are brief

and resulting anxiety can usually be alleviated by supportive reassurance.

Withdrawal from Multiple Drugs

Multiple sedative-hypnotics. Individuals withdrawing from several
sedative-hypnotic drugs, often including alcohol, are best managed by substituting one, long-acting sedative-hypnotic and following a taper procedure such as described in detoxification from
sedative-hypnotic drugs, above.

Sedative-hypnotics and opioids or stimulants. As a general rule, it
is best to treat the sedative hypnotic withdrawal first. Sedative-
hypnotic withdrawal represents the most medically risky and difficult process. When the "other" drug is one or more opioids,
the opioid may be stabilized with oral methadone or codeine
while the sedative-hypnotic is tapered, beginning opioid detoxification once the sedative-hypnotic substitute is completely withdrawn. Clonidine has been suggested as an adjunctive to this
process in that it alleviates withdrawal symptoms for both drug
groups.

■ MEDICAL MANAGEMENT OF DUAL-DIAGNOSIS PATIENTS

The medical management of persons with a dual diagnosis of drug
addiction and psychiatric disorders requiring medication poses
both conceptual and clinical problems. Although psychoactive
medications are helpful when properly used, patients with a personal or family history of substance abuse have a high risk for compulsively using all psychoactive drugs, and these drugs should
not be prescribed for them. The question is, what is the appropriate
medical response to a person who has addictive disease, or a
genetic pre-disposition to addictive disease, but who is otherwise
a good candidate for psychoactive medications? Clearly, physicians must use different prescribing standards for patients with
addictive disease and for the general population.

It is in the best interest of patients with both addictive disease
and psychiatric problems to first seek non-psychoactive therapy

alternatives, such as: non-psychoactive drugs, acupuncture, exercise, biofeedback, and other stress reduction techniques for the alcoholic patient with anxiety. When the severity of the psychiatric problem limits the person's ability to function, and if the use of non-psychoactive drug alternatives fails, then psychoactive drugs may need to be administered. Unfortunately, these patients will probably then develop compulsivity for the medications, lose control over them, and continue using them in spite of adverse consequences. The physician must exercise the utmost of caution in prescribing for these cases. The fundamentals of good prescribing practices can be thought of as the "six Ds," i.e., diagnosis, dosage, duration, discontinuation, dependence, and documentation.

Physicians make good-faith diagnoses of patients' problems. For an acute problem, such as a brief episode of pain or anxiety, it is within the accepted standard of care to treat that problem based on a tentative diagnosis. As an acute problem lingers and becomes chronic, a firm diagnosis must be made. Because anxiety, insomnia, and pain are invisible disorders, physicians must take the time to find the etiology of the problem.

Once the diagnosis has been made, and a treatment plan outlined, the physician can select the drug that is clinically indicated for the specific problem, prescribing the appropriate drug dosage for the diagnosis, and tailoring the medication schedule to the patient. The treatment goal is to neither undermedicate nor overmedicate, and as symptom severity increases and decreases, the medication should likewise be increased and decreased.

The duration of drug treatment should be planned with the patient, and medication should not be provided in an open-ended fashion. Also, periodic evaluations should be conducted to determine whether the medication should be discontinued: Are there problems with the drug? Has the planned duration of use expired? Has the crisis or problem that prompted use of the drug diminished or disappeared? Has the patient learned alternative ways of dealing with the original problem?

During treatment, the patient should be carefully monitored for developing dependence and toxicity problems. Physicians have a legal and ethical duty to warn the patient about both the side effects of the medications and the potential for developing dependence—which, for a person with addictive disease, can trigger an episode of compulsively taking prescribed and other drugs.

Finally, it is critical to carefully document the patient's initial complaints, eventual diagnosis, course of treatment, and all pre-scriptions and consultations. Consultations with experts in allied fields can be useful to the primary care physician. Addiction spe-cialists can be consulted for cases of addiction and dependence, much as one would consult a pain specialist or a psychiatrist. These consultations and decisions based on them should also be documented in the patient's file.

The Changing Face of Treatment

In the 1960s, when drug treatment first began to emerge from the criminal justice system, there were two primary approaches to treatment. Street-front clinics and hospital units still followed the Lexington/Fort Worth concept that treatment was synonymous with detoxification. Detoxification could be accomplished through social model programs that offered counseling and support for the addict during withdrawal, or medical models that provided symp-tomatic medication or other medical means of easing the addict's withdrawal symptoms. Therapeutic communities provided longer-term living support even after withdrawal. A third approach, opioid agonist maintenance, came with the approval of methadone.

As time passed, it became clearer that detoxification, in and of itself was not the whole story. As the treatment community absorbed lessons from the recovering community, i.e., that recov-ery is a lifelong process, it saw itself increasingly as the bridge between active addiction and active recovery. As a catalyst for change, treatment involves a highly complex and interactive pro-cess that will be dealt with in the second half of this book. Medical and behavioral therapies are not independent from each other, but in the best of circumstances represent an interdependent approach to helping addicts create a new life for themselves that has meaning in and of itself without the use of drugs.

One aspect is that of coming to terms with craving. Craving can be seen as a mixture of brain chemistry and culture, drug reaction and learned response, all coming together to push the detoxified and hopefully recovering addict back toward active use. What can be done about it?

■ ADVANCES IN THE TREATMENT OF CRAVING

Many important breakthroughs are being made in the treatment of addiction, and in the forefront of these are advances in the development of anti-craving agents. Anti-craving agents play an important role in the transition from acute drug abuse treatment into aftercare, abstinence, and recovery.

As a result of both scientific developments and the increasing interaction between medicine and the recovery community, treatment for addiction to alcohol and other drugs is getting better and the long-term outcome statistics are improving. Addiction medicine, as the study and treatment of addictive disease, has evolved from a medical pariah in the 1960s to status as a dynamic medical specialty, represented at the American Medical Association and having its own specialty organization, the American Society of Addiction Medicine (ASAM) in the 1990s. There is now a worldwide addiction movement that owes its beginnings to pioneering efforts here in the United States.

Through science, the treatment field has learned much more about the nature of addiction. It is now known, for example, that addiction is a mid-brain phenomenon. Both denial and recovery are learned activities that involve the cerebral cortex, but addiction itself is within the province of the primitive brain.

Through Alcoholics Anonymous and the recovering community, the treatment field is learning that long-term abstinence and recovery are possible if the addict's craving can be kept at bay long enough for that individual to overcome denial and learn the process of recovery.

Regarding the roles of environment, genetics and predisposition in the development of addiction, it is our view that addiction equals genetics plus environment. Over time, anyone given high enough doses of a drug may become addicted to it. When a person has a genetic predisposition, or when use starts in early adolescence addiction happens sooner and with greater ease.

The importance of a family history of alcoholism and addiction in predicting vulnerability to addictive disease continues to be significant, while the spread of drug availability and use over the past few decades bears witness to the important role of environment. Today, there are an estimated 30–40 million chemically dependent individuals in the United States. In 1962, approximately 4 million people had been exposed to illicit drugs. By 1992, that figure had risen to over 80 million. There has also been a major increase in Axis I psychiatric disorder among young people.

In his *Divine Comedy,* Dante refers to the inhabitants of the lowest levels of hell as *those who yearn for what they most fear.* That is a good description of people suffering from addictive disease. Addiction is a disease that is characterized by compulsion, loss of control, and continued use in spite of adverse consequences. The disease is progressive and can be fatal if not treated, and it is fueled by craving "for what they most fear." In the 12-step world, it is said that one drink is too many, while a million are not enough. Alcoholics do not react to alcohol the way that non-alcoholics do. This is because, for the alcoholic, the first drink acts as a trigger, converting craving into an overwhelming need for alcohol. The mechanisms of craving are not clearly understood, but the dynamic seems to hold true for those addicted to cocaine, heroin, tobacco, and other drugs as well as for alcohol.

Tobacco is specifically included in the above list to counter the perception that, with the exception of alcohol, addiction medicine only deals with illicit drugs. Much is being done within the addiction medicine field to promote awareness of tobacco addiction, and to enlist the primary-care physician in fighting it. Over 400,000 people a year die from smoking-related medical complications in the United States alone. Research is establishing that the action of nicotine in the human brain parallels that of cocaine. Tobacco companies even developed a form of nicotine freebase, but could not establish a market for their product. When the recognition of tobacco's deadly nature led to a decrease in adult smokers, the industry launched a massive advertising campaign targeting young people. Consequently, use of tobacco by adolescents is skyrocketing, and Joe Camel is as well known to children as Micky Mouse. The increasing use of tobacco by adolescents is particularly frightening in that smoking and drinking have been recognized as the primary indicators of future drug use. In view of all this, it is critical that the primary-care physician be educated as to the nature of addictive disease and its particular threat, via alcohol and tobacco, to adolescent patients. Drug abuse is occurring in a younger and younger population, and it is often the best and the brightest young people who succumb to addiction.

Obviously, drug presence, abuse, and addiction are on the rise, especially among adolescents, but why is it that drugs have such a profound effect? How are psychoactive substances capable of producing addiction, even among the most creative and intelligent individuals? The overall process involves two different areas in the human brain. While denial and recovery take place in the cerebral cortex, addiction and craving are activities of the more primitive mid-brain. Denial can be combated and recovery engendered through psychosocial treatment that involves counseling and the development of a program of supported recovery, such as that found in 12-Step fellowships, but these efforts are frequently sabotaged by the powerful fundaments of addiction, including craving, that lie inaccessible to reason within the mid-brain. It is in making it possible for psychosocial treatment to take place that drug treatment medication, including anti-craving agents, become important adjuncts to treatment.

Medical interventions in drug abuse treatment are based on a variety of approaches and goals. In acute withdrawal and detoxification, medication goals may include withdrawal symptom suppression through symptomatic medication or drug replacement. Replacement and taper strategies are particularly important in detoxification from sedative-hypnotic drugs, such as alcohol and benzodiazepines, where there is a danger of potentially fatal seizure during withdrawal.

Other medications may work as neurotransmitter precursor loads, such as amino acid combinations. These are particularly helpful in the treatment for cocaine abuse, in that cocaine exhausts several neurotransmitters in the brain. As these neurotransmitters are replenished, however, craving for cocaine becomes stronger. Anti-craving agents usually come into use once acute withdrawal is over and detoxification has been successfully completed. Essentially, the brain is like a chemical symphony of inhibitory and stimulatory neurotransmitters. Addiction disrupts this symphony. Recovery rebalances the brain and medications help in the process of rebalancing.

Anti-craving agents work in a variety of ways to reduce midbrain craving. Craving is not the absence of will, therefore the exercise of will is not a viable means of eliminating craving. Many individuals need help to avoid the overpowering urge to use so that they can participate in the forms of psychosocial treatment utilized in post-detoxification aftercare.

There is a high dropout rate of patients early in drug abuse treatment. Often this occurs shortly after detoxification. Patients rarely come into treatment to become fully abstinent. They come in because their lives are a mess and their use is totally out of control. As soon as things start coming together for them, the craving for their drug of choice returns, and if unchecked, will lead them out of treatment and back into active addiction. Anti-craving agents will bolster whatever desire they may have to stay in treatment, providing an extended window of opportunity for the treatment to be reinforced and hopefully take effect in leading them beyond their "need" for the drug.

One of the earliest anti-craving agents is disulfiram, usually known as anabuse. Ideally, anabuse reduces desire for alcohol by nullifying the desired reward payoff. It works by blocking the metabolization of an alcohol metabolite, acetaldehyde, in the liver. Acetaldehyde is particularly toxic, and its buildup causes acute discomfort for anyone who drinks alcohol while they are being maintained on anabuse. Unfortunately, if the urge to drink is too great, the user may try to override the anabuse acetaldehyde reaction with alcohol and become seriously ill in the process.[22]

A primary anti-craving agent for heroin and other opioid abusers is naltrexone. Naltrexone is an opioid antagonist. It works by actually blocking the endogenous morphine receptor sites in the brain that are utilized by opioids. Naltrexone is not psychoactive, so when it occupies the opioid receptor sites it produces no drug effect. One dose of naltrexone will continue to occupy these sites for up to 72 hours. If a user who is being maintained on naltrexone uses heroin or another opioid drug, nothing will happen. The opioid drug cannot engage the brain receptor sites, so it circulates harmlessly in the bloodstream until it is metabolized and excreted.

Carbamazapine and monoclonal antibodies and other new pharmacotherapy strategies are being tested experimentally for use as stimulant anti-craving agents. At present, however, there is no well-established cocaine or amphetamine anti-craving agent. Stimulant drugs cause massive disruption of brain chemistry. A pilot study is in progress for the use of naltrexone as an anti-craving agent for cocaine treatment. The National Institute on Drug Abuse should have results on that study in about 3 years.

One of the most promising anti-craving agents for alcohol craving is naltrexone, approved by the Food and Drug Administration for that indication in 1995 and currently marketed as Revia®. This is the same naltrexone that has proved effective in opioid addiction aftercare as an opioid antagonist. Clinical observation suggests that when naltrexone is used to block opioid receptor sites, it also decreases craving for opioid drugs. According to several recent studies[23,24] naltrexone would appear to decrease craving for alcohol as well.

In the Volpicelli study,[24] 70 male alcohol-dependent patients participated in a 12-week, double-blind placebo-controlled trial of naltrexone hydrochloride as an adjunct to aftercare treatment following detoxification from alcohol. Those subjects who took the naltrexone hydrochloride (50 mg/d) reported significantly less alcohol craving. Over the course of the study, only 23% of the naltrexone-treated subjects relapsed, compared to 54.3% in the placebo control group. The most significant effect, however, was seen in the patients who drank during the study period. Of the placebo subjects, 19 (95%) out of 20 relapsed after sampling alcohol, while only 8 (50%) of 16 naltrexone-treated subjects exposed to alcohol met relapse criteria.

Alcoholism, as is true with any addictive disease, is a chronic condition often marked by slips and relapses. Continuity in the treatment process and the development of long-term sobriety and recovery can best be accomplished when relapses are kept to a minimum. Slips often occur in the weeks following detoxification, and if these result in full relapse, the result can be devastating. The difference can be that between a single drink and full relapse with onset of pancreatitis. An agent utilized as an adjunct to treatment than can minimize the damage done by slips represents an important clinical aid to the treatment of addiction.

The study by Stephanie S. O'Malley, Ph.D., and her colleagues[23] involved 97 alcohol-dependent patients. Again, a 12-week, double blind, placebo-controlled format was used, utilizing two manual guided psychotherapies. Subjects were randomly provided either coping skills/relapse prevention therapy or a therapy designed to support the subjects' own coping skills. As in the former study, naltrexone proved superior to placebo in measures of drinking and alcohol-related problems, including abstention rates, number of drinking days, relapse, and severity of alcohol-related problems. As it turned out, the cumulative rate of abstinence was highest for patients treated with naltrexone and supportive therapy, while among the patients who initiated drinking, those who received naltrexone and coping skills therapy were the least likely to relapse.

In a subsequent study involving open-label usage assessment of more than 500 patients, nausea was seen to be a mild and transient nausea, seen in about 10%. Naltrexone has the capacity to cause liver toxicity at doses higher than recommended and should not be used in patients with active hepatitis or other liver disease. Adverse reactions seen in about 10% of patients include: difficulty sleeping, anxiety, nervousness, abdominal pain/cramps, nausea/vomiting, low energy, joint and muscle pain, and headache.[25] Long-term use of naltrexone in the treatment of opioid addiction has shown it to be non-habit forming and not a drug of abuse.

Clinical protocols recently developed and adopted by the Haight Ashbury Free Clinics Drug Detoxification, Rehabilitation, and Aftercare program recommend that naltrexone (Revia®) may be used in the aftercare treatment of alcohol abuse and addiction. Patients eligible for adjunct treatment with naltrexone should meet the DSM-IV criteria for alcohol dependence and have 5–7 days abstinence from alcohol (as well as 7–10 days abstinence from opioid drugs) and not be in active withdrawal. Naltrexone therapy is contraindicated for patients with acute hepatitis or liver failure (or exhibiting SGPT, SGOT levels at three times normal and who have elevated bilirubin levels), current use of opioids, or engaged in acute opioid withdrawal. No adequate studies have been done on the safety of naltrexone in pregnancy or in pediatric use. After an initial dosage of 25 mg/d, the patient can be maintained at 50 mg/d for a 3-month trial period. If the therapy seems to be of help and there are no adverse reactions, treatment can continue with re-evaluation every 3 months. Although use of naltrexone in alcohol treatment is relatively new, it has been used for years at a time in the aftercare treatment of opioid addicts without notable adverse effects.

PART II: PHARMACOLOGICAL AND BEHAVIORAL THERAPIES

In Part I of this chapter, the authors dealt with the beginnings of addiction treatment: care for acute intoxication and treatment of withdrawal or detoxification. For a large part of the 20th century, and in the aftermath of the Harrison Narcotic Act, these two represented what there was of treatment for alcoholism and other forms of drug addiction. A further step was initiated—one could say a further 12 Steps were initiated—in 1935 by alcoholics/

addicts themselves with the formation of Alcoholics Anonymous, of which much more will be said in Chapter 7.

After World War II, addiction treatment branched into two paths with the medical development of methadone maintenance and the beginnings of the therapeutic community social model approach. Other approaches followed, such as the combined medical social model outpatient and inpatient treatment programs and the use of counseling in combination with non-narcotic, symptomatic medication adopted by many free and community clinics. In general, addiction treatment has an overall goal of serving as a bridge between active addiction and active abstinence and recovery. Today, most medical treatment protocols combine elements of pharmacological therapies and behavioral therapies, and addiction medicine specialists are aware that a combination of approaches is needed to get the job done.

In the process of treating addiction, it is important to remember that addictive disease is a *chronic* condition and the addict is subject to slips and relapses both during and after treatment. A slip or relapse should not be a valid reason for terminating treatment. Every treatment episode is a window of opportunity for sowing the seeds of recovery and should be seen as such. Urinalysis is a good diagnostic tool, but a dirty urine in treatment should not be grounds for punishment. Instead, it should be a means of focusing and revising treatment as needed.

Pharmacological Therapies

■ TREATING OPIOID ADDICTION

Developing abstinence from chronic opioid abuse has been characterized as having two phases. The first, discussed in Part I, is acute withdrawal with all its attendant withdrawal symptoms. The second is a protracted abstinence syndrome that may continue for up to 6 months and include decreased blood pressure, decreased heart rate and body temperature, miosis and a decreased respiratory center sensitivity to carbon dioxide, as well as increased sedimentation rates and some EEG changes.[26]

Methadone assisted detoxification, which was discussed briefly in Part I of this chapter, can be seen as both a detoxification modality, and because of its protracted timing, as a pharmacological therapy as well. The taper can be seen as extending the detoxification and in the best of circumstances providing a longer window of opportunity for helping the patient make the transition from addictive thinking to recovery thinking.

Of longer duration is opioid agonist treatment (OAT) utilizing methadone and LAAM maintenance, currently involving some 115,000 of the estimated 600,000 opioid addicts in the United States. From a public health standpoint, in an era of spreading drug injection related disease such as AIDS and hepatitis-C, OAT provides a major harm and risk reduction service by reducing craving, preventing withdrawal, virtually eliminating the hazards of needle contamination, besides freeing the patient from the preoccupation of obtaining illegal opioids, enhancing ability to function and to utilize available psychosocial therapy.[27]

Methadone Maintenance

Methadone maintenance was first championed by Vincent Dole and Marie Nyswander in the 1960s.[28] Based on his clinical observations that opioid addicts develop a metabolic drive to return to active use, Dole saw methadone as a long-acting and controllable means of eliminating relapse and returning opioid addicts of productive non-criminal lives. As a maintenance drug used in agonist therapy, methadone had a distinct advantage over earlier protocols that utilized heroin, morphine, or other shorter-acting opioids. It could be administered orally, eliminating the use of hypodermic needles, it had a long half-life and could therefore be maintained on once-a-day dosage, and its use could be regulated and controlled. Steady-state levels can be reached after it is administered for 4–5 half-lives. With a half-life of 24–36 hours, a comfort zone can be maintained with once-a-day application.

Development of an affordable technology for measuring blood levels, combined with clinical documentation of the need for adequate methadone dosages to achieve positive outcome have in recent years improved treatment practices. In that there is no scientific or clinical basis for arbitrary dose ceilings on methadone or other agonist medication,[29] efforts to establish dose should be focused on achieving and maintaining a desired clinical response rather than adherence to arbitrary dose practices set by policy or regulation.

LAAM Maintenance

LAAM (levo-alpha-acetylmethadol) is a derivative of methadone that is capable of suppressing opioid withdrawal for over 72 hours. In all other ways, it is similar to methadone and can be administered every other day or 3 times weekly.

According to Payte and Zweben,[27] "Conversion from methadone to LAAM is simple, with the LAAM dose being 1.2 to 1.3 times the methadone dose given every 48 hours, with a 0–40% increase in LAAM dose for a 72-hour interval. At this time there are no provisions for a LAAM take-home dose, so daily methadone must be provided for emergencies, necessary travel, etc., at 80% of the 48-hour LAAM dose."

Maintenance with methadone, and more recently with LAAM has provided a relatively stable and regulatable basis for approved treatment within specialized centers licensed to that end. Such treatment, however, is limited in scope and limited to specialized providers. In an era of increased attention to the need for access to treatment for greater numbers of opioid addicts, new approaches that can be provided by non-addiction specialists in the health professions are being seriously considered. One of these is the utilization of buprenorphine.

Buprenorphine in Opioid Treatment

A partial agonist at the mu and kappa opioid receptors, Buprenorphine combines a strong receptor affinity with low intrinsic psychoactive activity and provides a high margin of safety and low chance of lethal overdose. Since the potential of buprenorphine in opioid addiction was first noted in the mid-1970s, there have been extensive clinical investigations for its use.[27]

Its general therapeutic effectiveness, high safety profile, patient acceptance, and relative ease of discontinuation make buprenorphine an ideal first medication for opioid dependence treatment, as illustrated in the diagram of sequential pharmacotherapeutic options following buprenorphine treatment.

As can be seen from Figure 6-1, patients successfully treated with buprenorphine have the option of going drug-free, with or without a period of treatment with naltrexone. Those patients with a level of dependence that cannot be adequately managed with buprenorphine can choose between LAAM and methadone and can be transferred between them according to both preference and treatment effectiveness.

Buprenorphine: Maintenance or Detoxification

Once the patient has been assessed, a diagnosis of opiate abuse or dependence made, and the potential benefits and risks of buprenorphine have been discussed with the patient, the next determination is whether maintenance or detoxification treatment meets the patient's current needs and goals. That decision can be revised depending on the patient's progress.

The objective of detoxification is to facilitate the patient's safe transition from a state of physical dependence on an opioid to an

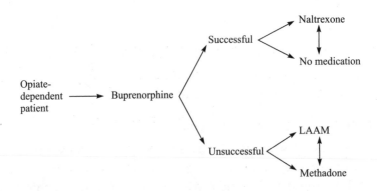

Figure 6-1 Sequential pharmacotherapeutic treatment of opioid dependence.

opioid-free state while minimizing withdrawal symptoms. The objective of buprenorphine maintenance is to substantially reduce or stop the use of illicit opioid drugs. The duration of maintenance will vary from patient to patient. After 6 months or more of abstinence from illicit opioids, the patient may consider tapering off maintenance if he or she has achieved changes sufficient to support recovery. Maintenance patients should be seen frequently in the early phase of treatment. Buprenorphine can be an aid to patients who are discontinuing methadone maintenance treatment.

Detoxification

The length of the detoxification period should be individualized to accommodate the patient's medical situation. The general strategy is to give gradually decreasing doses over time to allow reversal of physical dependence. Subsequent to this detoxification, an opiate antagonist (e.g., naltrexone) may be used as an adjunct to assist the patient in avoiding a recurrence of illicit opiate drug use. A physician interested in providing such treatment in an office setting will be required to take a certification course in prescribing and treating opioid-dependent patients. Local medical societies will be able to provide information on course location and presentation.

One needs to remember that opioid detoxification cannot be considered a complete treatment in itself. The goals of detoxification are mostly short-term and limited; they are to alleviate discomfort during opioid withdrawal and to provide an opportunity for the physician to diagnose concurrent, acute medical disease and to refer for other forms of treatment. Clinical consensus and available research data suggest that the majority of patients fail to complete detoxification or relapse shortly after completing the detoxification period. Nonetheless, detoxification has been accepted as an appropriate transitional treatment strategy in view of the danger of the spread of HIV and other infectious diseases associated with intravenous drug use. Potential patients should be informed of the high rate of failure and its accompanying danger and should receive information about additional or alternative treatment for opioid dependence, where it is available. Patients should not be denied detoxification if they refuse other treatment.[30]

Office-Based Treatment of Opioid Dependence

Because of the above qualities, buprenorphine may play an important role in office-based treatment of opioid addiction. Office-based treatment of opioid addiction is being considered as an option in various states where the need for treatment far outstrips the capacity of specialty treatment venues and there are long lists of individuals waiting for treatment slots to become available. There are concerns and considerations for the non-addiction specialist that have been addressed by the California Society of Addiction Medicine (CSAM) that are germane to this discussion.[30]

Special Patient Populations

Certain patients have special needs because of the complexity of their situation or diagnoses. They include those with concurrent alcohol or other substance abuse disorders, the psychiatrically ill, HIV+ patients, pregnant women, adolescents, and patients referred by the criminal justice system. Before accepting them for treatment of opioid dependence in an office setting, the physician should consider whether their needs can be met with the resources at hand in the office setting. If not, referral to a specialized treatment program should be considered.

Capacity to Get Urine Test Results

It is important to have a reliable system for collecting and testing urine collected either in your office or at a pre-arranged site. Shipment of urine samples for testing and turn around time for the results to be returned are also important issues that need to be satisfactorily resolved before undertaking office-based treatment of opioid dependence.

Be Hypersensitive to Being Conned

(A dictionary definition of "to con" is "to swindle by first gaining the victim's confidence.")

The usual admonition to avoid personal interaction with a patient deserves greater emphasis when treating addicts. Never have any personal dealings with a patient. This includes buying or selling things and lending money. If you do think a patient is in such dire straits that some help is needed, arrange to have someone in your office address the situation. Referral to ancillary sources of help and support should be considered.

At the same time that everyone on the treatment team should have a positive, accepting, non-judgmental, therapeutic attitude, they should be sensitive to the potential to be conned. Office procedures and treatment interactions should be structured as much as is feasible to avoid giving patients opportunities to steal or deceive.

Psychosocial Therapy in the Context of Office-Based Practice

For most patients, drug abuse counseling—individual or group—and participation in self-help programs such as Alcoholics Anonymous or Narcotics Anonymous are considered necessary, as pharmacotherapy alone is rarely sufficient treatment for drug dependency.

The ability to provide counseling and education within the context of private practice may vary considerably depending on the type and structure of the practice. Psychiatrists, for example, may include components of cognitive-behavioral therapy or motivational enhancement therapy during psychotherapy sessions. Some medical clinics may offer patient education, generally provided by allied health professionals such as nurse practitioners or physician assistants. A drug abuse treatment program includes counseling and drug abuse/HIV prevention education as an integral part of the clinic program. In a stand along general or family practice, the opportunities of education/counseling may be limited.

Where person-to-person teaching is limited, a patient "workbook" in printed form or videotape may be useful in conveying the core information that an opiate addict needs to know about buprenorphine and the recovery process. A set of questions covering the information patients should know may be useful for "self-assessment" and/or for assessing what kind of educational materials patients should be given.

Naltrexone: Agonist Maintenance in Opioid Dependence Treatment

Naltrexone is a long-acting opioid antagonist that provides complete blockage of opioid receptors then taken at least 3 times per week for a total weekly dose of about 350 mg.[31] As opposed to the agonist (methadone and LAAM) and agonist–antagonist (Buprenorphine) post-detox therapies discussed above, naltrexone blocks the reinforcing properties of opioid drugs by occupying the opioid receptors without providing any psychoactive effects. The action is similar to that of the short-acting naloxone used to reverse opioid overdose and discussed in the first half of this chapter. In essence, if the patient actively engaged in naltrexone maintenance were to slip and take an opioid, nothing would happen. Blocked from receptor sites, the opioid drug would circulate harmlessly and without effect in the bloodstream until it was metabolized and excreted.

Although naltrexone seems an ideal maintenance agent, and is, the greatest problem with maintenance is that of compliance. Because there is no narcotic effects, stopping use does not produce any withdrawal but leaves the addict open to opioid drug craving. Approaches to dealing with non-compliance can include family therapy and behavioral modification approaches. Individuals such as health-care professionals, pilots, business executives and probation referrals with a high stake in maintaining a drug-free recovery tend to have a higher compliance ratio. Also, an injectable, long-acting depot preparation that would eliminate the need for frequent doses is currently in development.[32] This long-acting preparation coupled with psychosocial therapy increases treatment compliance. Clinically the patient has to make a decision for abstinence once a month with the depot injection rather than once a day with the oral preparation.

Treatment with Naltrexone

Naltrexone maintenance should be initiated following opioid detoxification with at least a 5- to 7-day opioid-free period for short-acting opioids and a 7- to 10-day period for long-acting opioids. (It should be noted that in treatment cases involving detoxification mediated with a naltrexone/clonidine procedure the above does not apply.) The initial dose of naltrexone is generally 25 mg on the first day, followed by 50 mg daily or an equivalent of 350 mg weekly, divided into 3 doses (100, 100 and 150 mgs). The primary reason for a reduced dose on day 1 is the potential for GI side effects, such as nausea and vomiting, which occur in about 10% of cases. GI distress is relatively mild and transient in most cases, but it can be severe enough to warrant discontinuation of naltrexone treatment. Liver toxicity may occur; however, 50 mg daily has been given safely to opioid addicts.[33]

■ TREATMENT OF ALCOHOLISM AND OTHER SEDATIVE-HYPNOTIC DEPENDENCY

Alcohol

Given the social prevalence of alcohol in western culture—essentially world-wide culture these days—a major challenge in early recovery from alcohol abuse is that of providing relapse prevention. Much more will be said in the next chapter about the role of recovery fellowships in this matter. Here, the discussion turns to medical means of discouraging slips and relapses by the use of alcohol-sensitizing agents.

Sensitizing Agents[34]

While there are a variety of alcohol-sensitizing agents, the two most commonly in use are disulfiram and carbimide. These substances are similar in action. Both inhibit aldehyde dehydrogenase (ALDH). This is the enzyme that catalyzes oxidation of acetaldehyde, the primary metabolite of ethyl alcohol, into acetic acid. Acetaldehyde can be a very unpleasant metabolite when it builds up and not converted. The resulting symptoms can vary but they are always unpleasant.

Disulfiram (Antabuse®)

The disulfiram-ethanol reaction also varies in intensity depending on the amount of each substance in the system. Mild reactions can include warmth and flushing of the skin, increased heart rate, palpitations and lowered blood pressure, nausea, vomiting, shortness of breath, sweating dizziness, blurred vision and confusion, all lasting about 30 minutes. More severe reactions include marked tachycardia, hypotension, sometimes accompanied by bradycardia or cardiac arrest secondary to vagal stimulation from retching or vomiting, cardiovascular collapse, congestive failure and convulsions. Such severe reactions usually are associated with high doses of disulfiram (500 mg/day), combined with over 2 ounces of alcohol, but deaths have occurred at lower dosage and after imbibing a single drink.

The daily dosage of disulfiram has been limited in the United States to between 250 and 500 mg/day. It is usually administered orally. Implant dosages have been developed but produce blood levels too low to exert alcohol-sensitizing effects in most cases. Antabuse works best when it blocks opportunistic use while the individual works his or her psychosocial program, e.g., Antabuse + A.A. works better than Antabuse alone.

Calcium Carbimide (Temposil®)

Carbimide reactions are generally milder than those produced by disulfiram, and the half-life is much shorter. Usually, a 50 mg dose is administered twice a day. The short duration lends itself to use on an intermittent basis, i.e., when the patient is going to be in a situation where alcohol may be served and present a temptation to use. In use in Europe and Canada, carbimide is not available in the United States.

■ GENERAL COMMENTS

Why, one may ask, would anyone risk these symptoms after being prescribed disulfiram. Why indeed? For many patients disulfiram or Anabuse® is a powerful deterrent to ever touching alcohol. Yet, the disease and alcohol craving can be strong enough to lead some patients to ignore the discomfort and dangers and drink anyway. Clearly, the greatest value of alcohol sensitizers is the deterrent effect. They should never be employed as the only treatment, given the potentially dire consequences of actually using alcohol while these drugs are in one's system. The practitioner must be sensitive to the danger and only prescribe when doing so should have the desired deterrent effect.

■ REDUCING ALCOHOL CONSUMPTION THROUGH ALTERING BRAIN CHEMISTRY

The action of alcohol in the brain is highly complex, involving several neurotransmitter systems. These include the endogenous opioids, catecholamines, serotonin, and certain amino acids. Treatment based on the premise of working within these systems appears promising, but in most cases is still in the experimental realm with efficacy experienced under certain circumstances but as yet unproved.

Endogenous Opioid Systems

Because alcohol works within the endogenous opioid system, naltrexone has proved efficacious in reducing craving and relapse among alcoholics when its use was combined with psychosocial therapy.[35,36] However, the same problems with compliance have been seen as are experienced with its use in opioid treatment. A further problem with naltrexone maintenance treatment is the potential for hepatotoxicity. At a time when Hepatitis C is emerging as a widespread co-factor in addiction, care must be taken to complete liver workups prior to administration and to perform periodic liver function examinations.

Catecholaminergic Systems

Animal studies suggest that adrenergic systems are involved in the reinforcing effects of ethanol. Horwitz and colleagues found that the beta blocker atenolol decreased drinking desire,[37] although further studies have yet to confirm this.

The dopamine system also appears to be involved in alcohol addiction. Bromocriptine, a dopamine agonist, appears to be helpful in reducing craving and relapse.

Serotonergic Agents

Similarly, a variety of selective serotonin reuptake inhibitors (SSRIs) have undergone human tests to determine their effects on alcohol consumption and may reduce drinking in non-depressed, heavy drinkers but not by great magnitude.

Acamprosate® (calcium acetylhomotaurinate), an amino acid derivative has shown some promise in affecting both gamma-aminobutyric acid (GABA) and excitatory amino acid neurotransmission and thereby reducing the rate of return to drinking.

In summing this up, the most promising agents for directly reducing alcohol consumption are naltrexone and acamprosate. More research is needed, however, to determine when and why they are most efficacious—including which patient groups, dosage schedules, duration of therapy and concomitant psychosocial treatments are optimal for their use.

Post-Withdrawal Affective Disturbances

For many alcoholics in early recovery, the acute withdrawal syndrome may merge into a post-withdrawal state, often characterized by a continuation of the anxiety, insomnia, and general distress that occur in acute withdrawal but may last for weeks or months. While some of the symptoms may be "protracted withdrawal," others may be symptoms of emerging co-morbid psychiatric disorders. Kranzler and Jaffe[34] identify 7 factors that may have a causal role in problems during the post-withdrawal period:

1. heavy alcohol intake;
2. acute and protracted withdrawal;
3. alcohol-induced CNS damage;
4. CNS damage from indirect effects of alcohol (e.g., head trauma, thiamine deficiency);
5. social, economic, and interpersonal losses;

6. antecedent psychiatric disorders; and
7. a cluster of signs and symptoms that may be referred to as the "defeat/depression/ hypophoria cluster."

Comorbid Disorders

The most common comorbid disorders found in post-withdrawal alcoholics are: major depression, bipolar disorder, anti-social personality disorder, phobias, and hyperactivity syndrome residual type attention deficit disorder.

Treatment of Comorbid Disorders

Drugs that have been used to treat post-withdrawal state anxiety and depression include: tricyclic antidepressants, selective serotonin reuptake-inhibiting antidepressants, benzodiazepines and other anxiolytics, phenothiazines and other dopaminergic blockers, and lithium. Care should always be taken in prescribing medications for alcoholics so as to take into account an increased potential for negative drug interactions in this population. Disulfiram, for example, may interact negatively with a variety of medications used to treat psychiatric disorders. If the patient relapses into acute or chronic alcohol consumption, there is the danger of pharmacokinetic effects. For example, chronic ethanol use will increase clearance of imipramine and desipramine, reducing their therapeutic potential. A potentially fatal synchronistic effect can occur if a patient uses alcohol while being treated with benzodiazepines or other sedative-hypnotic drugs.

Any practitioner who is treating alcoholics with post-withdrawal complications should become familiar with the most up-to-date information on any medications contemplated. This is not to say that treatment personnel should avoid treating comorbid conditions. Unless the condition is a direct result of ethanol abuse, it will not simply go away in the course of recovery and if ignored may be a cause of continued misery and potential relapse into active addiction for the patient.

Educating the Patient, and the Recovering Community

Another possible concern involves the patient's interaction within the recovering community. Although there is increasing education, including A.A. pamphlets that discuss the need for medicating certain conditions in recovery, there are still well-meaning individuals within the recovering community who are convinced that any use of psychoactive materials, including prescribed medications, is antithetical to recovery. There have been too many instances of great harm, including death resulting from patients being convinced by fellows in recovery that they should flush their medications down the toilet in order to be fully drug-free. While it may be impossible to educate every recovery meeting that a patient may attend, counseling on this topic and some monitoring may be needed to counteract such persuasion.

■ TREATMENT FOR SEDATIVE-HYPNOTIC DRUG ADDICTION

Much of the addiction to benzodiazepines and other sedative-hypnotic drugs is either iatrogenic, resulting from treatment with these drugs for a variety of disorders, or from attempts at self-medication. Benzodiazepine dependence differs from most other drug addictions because, aside from the sedating and some degree of disinhibition, these drugs produce few desirable mood-altering effects. Most patients develop sedative-hypnotic dependence while they are being treated for anxiety disorders or insomnia. Others may be stimulant or opioid abusers who became dependent while using black-market sedative-hypnotics to self-medicate symptoms produced by other drugs.[38] In that self-medication is a recurring theme with sedative-hypnotics, most of these patients have underlying disorders that must be addressed.

With the exception of alcohol, discussed above, sedative-hypnotics are rarely primary drugs of abuse and are not taken daily to produce intoxication. There are, however, exceptions.

Treatment strategies for sedative-hypnotic dependence cannot be separated from the realities of current health-care delivery. Physicians often find themselves in the position of having to devise not the optimal treatment plan, but one that can be negotiated with the patient and the payer. The realities of today's fractured health-care dictate rethinking pharmacological treatment strategies for sedative-hypnotic dependence. Health-care payers and the agents of managed care may have simplistic and unrealistic criteria for assigning patients to level of care. (ASAM's Patient Placement Criteria—included as an appendix to this book—are clinically derived and should be followed whenever possible.) Some—if not most—of the assessment and treatment of sedative-hypnotic dependence thus must be accomplished on an outpatient basis. The assessment and treatment of physical dependence is more complex for the physician and carries more risk for the patient on an outpatient than on an inpatient basis. In an inpatient setting, the patient's access to medications can be better controlled, the patient's response to medications can be closely observed, and the patient is not tempted to drive an automobile while experiencing toxicity or withdrawal symptoms.

The uncertainties associated with outpatient management of withdrawal can be reduced by establishing clear goals, employing a systematic assessment procedure, and devising a clearly defined treatment protocol. Assessment and treatment protocols help the physician to systematically accumulate the information needed to initiate treatment and monitor treatment progress. Well-structured assessment and treatment protocols are also useful in negotiating with treatment payers and managed care entities around payment for the treatment the patient needs. Detailed medical records can be important in documenting the patient's clinical course and adverse events, and can buttress the physician's argument for a more intensive level of care when needed.[38]

Post-Withdrawal Treatment

Withdrawal from sedative-hypnotic drugs is usually successful when the patient cooperates, but many patients do not remain abstinent. For patients with an underlying anxiety disorder, relapse may mean that the patient is unable or unwilling to tolerate the symptoms that emerge following detoxification. For patients with a dual diagnosis, outcomes other than drug abstinence must be considered. Fortunately, there are now pharmacological alternatives to benzodiazepines and the older sedative-hypnotics for treatment of anxiety. In addition, cognitive-behavioral therapies and other psychotherapeutic and behavioral treatments for anxiety have shown efficacy.

Detoxification alone is not adequate treatment for sedative-hypnotic dependence, but rather the first step in the recovery process. Adjunctive use of medications such as carbanazepine, imipratime, and buspirone have been found to result in significantly higher discontinuation rates.

Because of its low abuse potential and benign side effects, buspirone would seem a likely candidate for continuation. Buspirone appears to act as a serotonin HT1A partial agonist.[39] There is, however, some suggestion that patients with a history of benzodiazepine abuse are resistant to the anxiolytic effects of buspirone, and it does not appear to be efficacious in managing panic disorders or social phobias. It may be particularly useful as an alternative to benzodiazepines for managing anxiety in elderly patients who are vulnerable to the cognitive impairment related to benzodiazepine use. In general, supportive individual psychotherapy or self-help recovery group support is needed as part of the recovery plan for patients who have a sedative-hypnotic substance abuse disorder.

■ TREATING COCAINE AND OTHER STIMULANT ADDICTIONS

Pharmacological therapies for cocaine and other stimulant addicts are in a general state of development. At present, there is a lack of consensus on effective pharmacotherapy, in which at least 15 different medications have been reported to be in use by addiction medicine practitioners, despite their own doubts about effectiveness.[40]

In general, the treatment goals for cocaine and other stimulants are essentially the same as those for other modalities, i.e., to help patients abstain and to regain control over their lives. Mechanisms suggested for accomplishing this by Gorelick[40] are:

1. reducing or eliminating the positive reinforcement from taking a cocaine or other stimulant dose;
2. reducing or eliminating a subjective state that predisposes to taking cocaine, such as craving;
3. reducing or eliminating negative reinforcement from taking a cocaine dose (as by reducing withdrawal-associated behavior;
4. making cocaine-taking aversive; or
5. increasing the positive reinforcement obtained from non-cocaine taking behaviors.

The medications that are currently available are thought to act by one or more of the first three. The fourth mechanism, which would be equivalent to the use of Anabuse® (disulfiram) for alcoholics, has no counterpart for stimulants. The fifth is currently served by psychosocial treatment.

Again according to Gorelick,[40] there are at least four potentially useful pharmacological approaches to stimulant treatment. These are:

1. substitution treatment with a cross-tolerant stimulant (analogous to methadone maintenance treatment of opiate addiction);
2. treatment with an antagonist medication that blocks the binding of cocaine at its site of action (true pharmacological antagonism, analogous to naltrexone treatment of opiate addiction);
3. treatment with a medication that functionally antagonizes the effects of stimulants (e.g., reduces the reinforcing effects of or craving for cocaine);
4. alteration of drug metabolism to either enhance its elimination from the body or change its metabolic profile (analogous to disulfiram treatment of alcoholism).

Among the medications that have been cited in stimulant abuse treatment are: antidepressants, particularly desipramine and other heterocyclic antidepressants; selective serotonin reuptake inhibitors (SSRIs); monoamine oxidase (MAO) inhibitors;

dopamine agonists, such as bromocriptine and mantadine; less harmful stimulants used analogous with methadone maintenance treatment of opiate addiction; neuroleptics; anti-convulsants; amino acids; lithium; calcium channel blockers; and combinations of the above.

In surveying the data, Gorelick[40] concludes that: The failure of existing medications to show consistent efficacy in the treatment of cocaine (and other stimulant) addiction has prompted growing interest in pharmacokinetic approaches, i.e., preventing ingested cocaine from entering the brain and/or enhancing its elimination from the body. The former could be implemented by active or passive immunization to produce binding antibodies which keep cocaine from crossing the blood-brain barrier. The latter could be implemented by administration of the enzyme (butyrylcholinesterase) which catalyzes cocaine hydrolysis or by immunization with a catalytic antibody. The pharmacokinetic approaches have shown promise in attenuating cocaine's effects in animals, but have not yet been studied in humans.

■ MARIJUANA

There are a variety of drugs for which there are no recognized or proven role for medication in treatment. Among these are marijuana, although a specific receptor site has been identified, creating the possibility of future use of a synthetic antagonist to block the effects of cannabis. Such an antagonist has been developed and appears to block the effects in animals. The compound, listed as SR 141716A, is in Phase 1 human trials.

■ ANABOLIC STEROIDS

Adjunctive pharmacological treatment can be helpful in combating steroid-induced violence and aggressive behavior, steroid-induced depression, and detoxification via tapering doses of steroid medications. Low-dose neuroleptics (e.g., phenothiazine-equivalent doses of about 200 mg/day) have been effective for psychosis, hostility and agitation, while tricyclic antidepressants may exacerbate psychological symptoms.

■ CAFFEINE

Although the DSM-IV does not recognize it, a caffeine withdrawal syndrome does exist and it can contribute to relapse for those who are plagued with caffeine sensitivity, or who have a use pattern that is out of control, or who need to stop. In general, withdrawal symptoms may begin about 19 hours after last use, peak in the first 48 hours and resolve within a week.[41] There is no viable substitute to offset withdrawal or decrease craving, therefore, tapered withdrawal is the pharmacological treatment of choice. A suggested 6-day taper based on an individual who drinks six cups of coffee per day is as follows: 1st day: 5 cups caffeinated coffee/1 cup decaffeinated, decreasing caffeinated and increasing decaffeinated 1 cup per day to 6th day: no cups caffeinated/6 decaffeinated. For patients with severe dependence, caffeine pills can be used. Treatment should include patient education about the adverse consequences of chronic caffeine use and the variety of products and medications containing caffeine. Increased water intake and sugarless mints have been suggested to help alleviate craving.

■ HALLUCINOGENS AND PHENCYCLIDINE (PCP)

A variety of medications have been tried with hallucinogens with mixed results. As with cannabis, it can be said that there are no currently available pharmacological treatments for hallucinogen abuse.[42] The same is true for phencyclidine and ketamine.

■ INHALANTS

There are no pharmacological treatments for the addiction to this heterogeneous group of substances that include adhesives, aerosols, anesthetics, gasoline, cleaning agents, food products, paint and room odorizers, in fine, many different chemical agents with a wide variety of properties, effects, and toxicities. Treatment is primarily psychosocial, conducted in a supportive, non-confrontational atmosphere, and directed toward developing basic social and personal skills. Inpatient treatment is recommended when there is severe psychiatric sequelae or use cannot be otherwise controlled. Given the neurologic and hepatic toxicity of chronic inhalant use, a thorough medical evaluation should be made at the start of treatment.

■ TREATING NICOTINE DEPENDENCE

With the increasing recognition of the deadly nature of nicotine dependence—roughly 400,000 people in the United States alone die each year from nicotine-related illness—treatment of nicotine addiction has developed rapidly. The most widely used and accepted pharmacological treatment of nicotine addiction involves using nicotine itself as an agonist drug replacement in nicotine replacement therapy (NRT).[43] In NRT, the dependent smoker is provided with a form of nicotine delivery that provides some of the pharmacological effects of smoking or chewing with lower abuse liability. This includes slower entry into the brain than that found with smoking. Present vehicles for NRT include: nicotine polacrilex marketed as Nicorette® gum with 2 or 4 mg nicotine bound to an ion-exchange resin and gum base; transdermal nicotine patches; nicotine nasal spray; and nicotine inhaler, a "puffer" containing a cartridge with 10 mg nicotine and 1 mg menthol, approved by the FDA in 1997.

Each of these NRTs has been effective in reducing withdrawal symptoms and improving abstinence outcomes. The best results, however, have come from combining NRT treatment with behavioral therapy so as to address environmental coping skills.

Psychosocial/Behavioral Therapies

Every pharmaceutical treatment intervention for addiction comes with the caveat that it can be effective only when combined with some form of psychosocial therapy. Addiction is a disease that effects not only the physical being but the spiritual and psychological being as well. If treatment is to be the bridge between active addiction and active recovery, it needs to be more than just treatment of withdrawal symptoms and biological rebalancing. Counseling and related therapies are the key to successful spiritual and psychological treatment, preparing the addicted patient for a lifetime of recovery.

Counseling takes many forms. When drug treatment first emerged from the punitive criminal-justice systems prevalent in the post-World War II decades, there were no trained drug counselors. Spiritual support was primarily for the fortunate alcoholics who found their way into Alcoholics Anonymous where they found "sponsors" among the alcoholics who were already in the fellowship. When drug treatment became available, the store-front clinics and therapeutic communities who were the providers drew their counseling staffs from the only population that understood addiction, recovering or at least detoxified addicts.

In the 1970s, steps began toward education and certification for alcohol and other drug abuse counselors. The Career Teachers Program, initiated by the National Institute on Mental Health, provided training for medical students in drug abuse treatment. Various states initiated certification programs, and as insurance began covering drug treatment in the 1980s, alcohol and other drug abuse counseling became a career destination rather than a post-detoxification activity. Colleges and universities established their own credential programs. State-wide entities, such as CAADAC in California, set certification standards for their members. At the physician level, key individuals within pioneering state programs such as the California Society for the Treatment of Alcoholism and Other Drug Dependencies came together to form the American Society for the Treatment of Alcoholism and Other Drug Dependencies (AMSAODD). Changing its name with the coining of "addictionologists," the American Society of Addiction Medicine (ASAM) developed the addiction medicine specialty with the blessings of and membership within the American Medical Association (AMA) and proceeded to initiate educational and credentialing activities. ASAM's "diagnosis driven" criteria for both adults and adolescents are given in the appendices to this book.

■ A SPECTRUM OF THERAPIES

Today, there is a wide spectrum of therapists and psychosocial therapeutic approaches to drug abuse and addiction. Although education in the field has opened it to non-addict, non-recovering practitioners, the recovering addict who has received training in addiction treatment remains a major force in that spectrum, particularly in treatment settings where the ultimate goal is full abstinence and supported recovery. There is also a growing public health approach that advocates more modest goals in the interest of public safety, such as decreasing use and avoiding high-risk abuse and concomitant sexual activities.

Within general guidelines, there may be as many therapeutic approaches as there are therapists, with each adding a personal emphasis that may be based on training and personal experience. Given this variety, it is difficult to clearly ascertain what represents effective therapy and who is an effective therapist.

■ THERAPIST ATTRIBUTES AND CHARACTERISTICS

In ASAM's *Principles of Addiction Medicine,* Kathleen M. Carroll[44] points out that many studies have been conducted on the attributes of therapists and their impact on treatment but these have been contradictory and in sum inconclusive. While some studies cited by Carroll have suggested that therapists' age, gender, education and ethnicity are strongly related to treatment outcome, most have found no evidence of relation. Similarly, although a therapists recovery status is considered by many practitioners to be an important factor in treatment response, a review of 50 studies showed little correlation.[45] While there is evidence that other therapist attributes may contribute to improved treatment outcome. In general, a positive therapeutic relationship has been credited in improved outcome. Similarly, a directive, confrontational counselor style has been seen as associated with significantly more resistance by patients, producing a poorer 1-year outcome than that found from a more empathetic, client-centered style.[46] According to Carroll, "Another process variable that has been linked to improved patient outcomes is the therapist's level of adherence to a particular, well-defined treatment approach. This reflects the increased emphasis on careful specification of treatment delivery through the use of treatment manuals and the related emphasis on empirically validated treatment." She concludes that "Overall, effectiveness among therapists who deliver substance abuse treatment appears more closely related to what they do and how well they do it than to who they are."[44]

■ THERAPEUTIC GOALS: ENHANCING THE MOTIVATION TO CHANGE

Individuals rarely enter treatment with the desire to abstain from all psychoactive substance and begin a life-long program of supported recovery. Most often, they want help for a related health problem, or they have been remanded to treatment by the courts, or they are the victims of family, friends and/or business colleagues perceptions of their behavior. Increasingly, treatment may be initiated by family and/or colleagues through a more or less formal intervention, often with the guidance of a professional, staged so as the individual is entered into treatment immediately. A family physician or other health professional may also initiate a medical intervention when the abuse/addiction is suspected. Finally, the addict's place of business may initiate action by referring the individual to the company's Employee Assistance Program (EAP) for assessment.

The process of intervention involves not only a clear sense of the problem, but a motivating of the individual to take action as well. Prochaska[47] has enunciated the following set of principles to help motivate patients to progress from one stage to the next:

1. The benefits of change must increase before individuals will progress from pre-contemplation to contemplation.

2. The costs of change must decrease before individuals will progress from contemplation.

3. The relative balance between the benefits and costs of change must cross over for people to be prepared to take action.

4. The strong principle of progress holds that, to progress from pre-contemplation to effective action, the benefits of change must increase by one standard deviation.

5. The weak principle of progress holds that, to progress from contemplation to effective action, the costs of change must decrease by one-half standard deviation.

6. It is essential to match particular processes of change to specific stages of change.

The stages of change cited by Prochaska[47] include:

- *Consciousness raising*: increasing awareness about the causes, consequences and treatments.

- *Dramatic relief*: arousal (i.e., guilt, fear, inspiration and hope) around one's current behavior and the relief that can result from change.

- *Environmental reevaluation*: combination of affective and cognitive assessments of how addiction affects one's social environment and how changing it would effect that environment.

- *Self-reevaluation*: cognitive and affective assessment (involving such techniques as imagery, healthier role models, and values clarification) of one's self-image as it would be free from active addiction.

- *Self-liberation*: the belief that change is possible and the commitment and recommitment to act on that belief.

- *Counter-conditioning*: the learning of healthier behaviors that can replace addictive behavior.

- *Contingency management*: the systematic use of reinforcements and punishments through such means as contingency contracts, overt and covert reinforcements and group recognition for taking steps in the right direction. Emphasis on the positive wherever possible is recommended.

- *Stimulus control*: modifying environment to increase healthier response cues and decrease cues that undermine commitment to change.
- *Helping relationships*: developing dependence on such relationships as combine caring, openness, trust and acceptance, such as therapeutic alliance, counselor calls, buddy systems, sponsors and self-help groups.

■ BEHAVIORAL THERAPIES FOR ADDICTION

The American Society of Addiction Medicine's *Principles of Addiction Medicine* presents five broad categories of therapy: brief interventions, individual psychotherapy, network therapy, aversion therapy, and community reinforcement and contingency management interventions.

Brief Interventions

This category is the one that can most involve the primary-care physician who is in a position to identify a drug or alcohol use problem by viewing it along a continuum, rather than as a dichotomy between "addict" and "non-addict." This may be particularly true with the alcoholic where early stages of use are most likely social in nature. Utilizing such a continuum involves broadening one's focus to include both persons whose drinking patterns have just started to cause life problems and individuals with an increased risk of future problems, injury, or harm.[48]

In general, screening and brief intervention protocols should be routinely incorporated into primary medical care systems. Brief interventions have been used in two ways in health-care settings: as a stand-alone, self-help, self-guided strategy for changing drinking or drug use behavior, and as a referral strategy to motivate individuals to seek further help for their problems. In alcohol abuse, the former most suitable for non-dependent or risky drinkers, while the latter is most appropriate for dependent or severe problem drinkers.[48]

Individual Psychotherapy

Individual psychotherapy is most appropriate for patients who have a dual diagnosis of drug abuse/addiction and mental health problems as well. While the disease concept of addiction holds that addiction is a disease in and of itself rather than a symptom of underlying psychopathology, it is also true that a large percentage of alcohol and other drug addicts also suffer from mental illness. A team approach is recommended with such patients in which drug treatment and psychotherapy professionals work together to resolve the patient's multiple problems.

Network Therapy

Network therapy is a whole-systems approach. According to Galanter[49] the model of addictive behavior and office-based treatment involved deals with the influence of pharmacologically conditioned drinking cues on relapse into substance dependence, and it uses a cognitive-behavioral approach to averting relapse. "To engage addicted patients while treatment is applied and to motivate them to overcome the effect of addictive cues, a network of persons close to the patient can be brought into the therapy sessions to augment the individual treatment." Specific network techniques draw on the variety of relationships among the patient, the family and peers. (In that this approach touches directly on the physician's role in helping the patient into supported recovery, it will be covered more thoroughly in that context in the next chapter.)

Aversion Therapy

Aversion therapy is essentially counter-conditioning aimed at the part of the brain where emotional attachments are made or broken through experienced associations of pleasure or discomfort. It represents a means for helping the patient gain control over the use response to drug cues. Today there are a number of approaches, all of them with calculated risks and benefits.

Community Reinforcement and Contingency Management Interventions

According to Higgins and colleagues,[50] "...drug use is considered a normal, learned behavior that can be fruitfully conceptualized to fall along a continuum ranging from light use with no problems to heavy use with many untoward effects. The same basic learning processes are assumed to operate across the drug use continuum. Treatment strategies based on this conceptual framework look to weaken the reinforcement obtained from drug use and related activities and to enhance the material and social reinforcement obtained from other sources, especially from participation in activities deemed to be incompatible with a drug abusing lifestyle. Community reinforcement and contingency management procedures are based on this general strategy and have been demonstrated in controlled studies to be effective in treating alcohol, cocaine, and opioid dependence."

In the next chapter, we will be exploring the relationship between the practitioner, the patient and the community as represented by the various recovery programs and fellowships available to the addict. With the understanding that addiction is a chronic disease entity that cannot be cured but, like cancer and diabetes, potentially brought into lifelong remission, it can be seen that the health professional's role in furthering a meaningful and effective transition from treatment to recovery is of great importance to the spectrum of care.

REFERENCES

1. O'Brien CP, McLellan AT: Myths about the treatment of addiction, in: Graham AW, Schultz TK, Wilford BB (eds.), *Principles of Addiction Medicine,* 2nd ed. Chevy Chase, MD: American Society of Addiction Medicine, 1998, p. 309.
2. Musto D: *The American Disease: Origins of Narcotic Control,* expanded ed. New York, NY: Oxford University Press, 1987.
3. Hunt GH, Odoroff ME: Follow-up study of narcotic drug addicts after hospitalization. *Public Health Reports,* 1962; 77: 41–54.

4. O'Connor PG, Kosten TR: Management of opioid intoxication and withdrawal, in: Graham AW, Schultz TK, Wilford BB (eds.), *Principles of Addiction Medicine*, 2nd ed. Chevy Chase, MD: American Society of Addiction Medicine, 1998, p. 457.
5. Whipple JK, Quebbeman EJ, Lewis KS, Gottlieb MS, Ausman RK: Difficulties in diagnosing narcotic overdoses in hospitalized patients. *Annals of Pharmacotherapy*, 1994; 28(4): 446–50.
6. Eickelberg SJ, Mayo-Smith MF: Management of sedative-hypnotic intoxication and withdrawal, in: Graham AW, Schultz TK, Wilford BB (eds.), *Principles of Addiction Medicine*, 2nd ed. Chevy Chase, MD: American Society of Addiction Medicine, 1998, p.441.
7. Mayo-Smith MF: Management of alcohol intoxication and withdrawal, in: Graham AW, Schultz TK, Wilford BB (eds.), *Principles of Addiction Medicine*, 2nd ed. Chevy Chase, MD: American Society of Addiction Medicine, 1998, p. 431.
8. Wilkins JN, Conner BT, Gorelick DA: Management of stimulant, hallucinogen, marijuana and phencyclidine intoxication and withdrawal, in: Graham AW, Schultz TK, Wilford BB (eds.), *Principles of Addiction Medicine*, 2nd ed. Chevy Chase, MD: American Society of Addiction Medicine, 1998, p. 465.
9. Schuckit MA: *Drug and Alcohol Abuse: A Clinical Guide to Diagnosis and Treatment* 3rd ed. New York, NY: Plenum Publishing, 1989.
10. Wetli CV, Fisbain D: Cocaine-induced psychosis and sudden death. *Journal of Forensic Sciences*, 1985; 30: 873–80.
11. Callaway CW, Clark RF: Hyperthermia in psychostimulant overdose. *Annals of Emergency Medicine*, 1994; 24: 68–75.
12. Smith DE: Editor's Note. *Journal of Psychedelic Drugs*, 1967; 1(1): 1–5.
13. Smith DE, Seymour RB: Dream becomes nightmare: adverse reactions to LSD. *Journal of Psychoactive Drugs*, 1985; 17(4): 297–303.
14. Wesson DR, Smith DE: Psychedelics, in: Schecter A. (ed.), *Treatment Aspects of Drug Dependence*. West Palm Beach: CRC Press, 1975.
15. Seymour RB, Smith DE: *The Psychedelic Resurgence: Treatment, Support, and Recovery Options*. Center City: Hazelden, 1993.

16. Seymour RB, Smith DE: *Drugfree: A Unique, Positive Approach to Staying Off Alcohol and Other Drugs.* New York: Facts on File Publications, 1987.

17. Seymour RB: *MDMA.* San Francisco: Partisan Press, 1987.

18. Hayner GN, McKinney H: MDMA: the dark side of ecstasy. *Journal of Psychoactive Drugs,* 1986; 18(4): 341–347.

19. Giannini AJ, Loiselle RH, DiMarzio LR, Giannini MC: Augmentation of haloperidol by ascorbic acid in phencyclidine intoxication. *American Journal of Psychiatry,* 1987; 144: 1207–1209.

20. Tyrer P, Rutherford D, Hugett T: Benzodiazepine withdrawal symptoms and propanolol. *Lancet,* 1981; 1: 520–522.

21. Smith DE, Wesson DR (eds.): *The Benzodiazepines: Current Standards for Medical Practice.* Lancaster, England: MTP Press Limited, 1985.

22. Milam JR, Ketcham K: *Under the Influence: a Guide to the Myths and Realities of Alcoholism.* Seattle, WA: Madrona Publishers, Inc., 1981.

23. O'Malley SS, Jaffe AJ, Chang G, Schottenfeld RS, Meyer RE, Rounsaville B: Naltrexone and coping skills therapy for alcohol dependence: a controlled study. *Archives of General Psychiatry,* 1992; 49: 881–887.

24. Volpicelli JR, Alterman AI, Hayashida M, O'Brien CP: Naltrexone in the treatment of alcohol dependence. *Archives of General Psychiatry,* 1992; 49: 876-880.

25. Croop RS, Labriola DF, Wroblewski JM, Nibbelink DW: A multicenter safety study of naltrexone as adjunctive pharmacotherapy for individuals with alcoholism. Paper presented at the Annual Meeting of the American Psychiatric Association, Miami FL, May, 1995.

26. Martin WR, Jasinski DR: Physiological parameters of morphine dependence in man—tolerance, early abstinence, protracted abstinence. *Journal of Psychiatric Research,* 1969; 7: 9–17.

27. Payte JT, Zweben JE: Opioid maintenance therapies, in: Graham AW, Schultz TK, Wilford BB (eds.), *Principles of Addiction Medicine,* 2nd ed. Chevy Chase, MD: American Society of Addiction Medicine, 1998, p. 557.

28. Dole VP, Nyswander M: A medical treatment for diacetylmorphine (heroin) addiction—a clinical trial with methadone hydrochloride.

Journal of the American Medical Association, 1965; 193(8): 646–650.

29. Kaufman J, Payte JT, McLellan AT: Treatment standards and optimal treatment, in: Rettig RA, Yarmolinski A (eds.), *Institute of Medicine—Federal Regulation of Methadone Treatment.* Washington, DC: National Academy Press, 1995, pp. 185–216.

30. CSAM Committee on Treatment of Opioid Dependence: *Buprenorphine in Pharmacotherapy of Opioid Addiction: Implementation in Office-based Medical Practice: Translating the Experience of Clinical Trails into Clinical Practice.* Oakland, CA: California Society of Addiction Medicine, 1999.

31. Kosten TR, Kleber HD: Strategies to improve compliance with narcotic antagonists. *American Journal of Drug and Alcohol Abuse,* 1984; 10: 249–266.

32. Stine SM, Meandzija B, Kosten TR: Pharmacologic therapies for opioid addiction, in: Graham AW, Schultz TK, Wilford BB (eds.), *Principles of Addiction Medicine,* 2nd ed. Chevy Chase, MD: American Society of Addiction Medicine, 1998, p. 545.

33. Brahen LS, Capone TJ, Capone DM: Naltrexone: Lack of effect on hepatic enzymes. *Journal of Clinical Pharmacology,* 1988; 28: 64–70.

34. Kranzler HR, Jaffe JH: Pharmacologic therapies for alcoholism, in: Graham AW, Schultz TK, Wilford BB (eds.), *Principles of Addiction Medicine,* 2nd ed. Chevy Chase, MD: American Society of Addiction Medicine, 1998, p. 501.

35. Volpicelli JR, O'Brien C, Alterman A, Hayashida M: Naltrexone in the treatment of alcohol dependence. *Archives of General Psychiatry,* 1992; 49: 867–880.

36. O'Malley SS, Jaffe AJ, Chang G, Schottenfeld RS, Meyer RE, Rounsaville B: Naltrexone and coping skills therapy for alcohol dependence: a controlled study. *Archives of General Psychiatry,* 1992; 49, 894–898.

37. Horwitz RI, Kraus ML, Gottlieb LD: The efficacy of atenolol and the mediating effects of craving in the outpatient management of alcohol withdrawal. *Clinical Research,* 1987; 35: 348A.

38. Wesson DR, Smith DE, Ling W: Pharmacologic therapies for benzodiazepine and other sedative-hypnotic addiction, in: Graham AW, Schultz TK, Wilford BB (eds.), *Principles of Addiction Medicine,*

2nd ed. Chevy Chase, MD: American Society of Addiction Medicine, 1998, p. 517.

39. Taylor DP, Moon SL: Buspirone and related compounds as alternative anxiolytics. *Neuropeptides,* 1991; 19 (Suppl): 15–19.

40. Gorelick DA: Pharmacologic therapies for cocaine and other stimulant addiction, in: Graham AW, Schultz TK, Wilford BB (eds.), *Principles of Addiction Medicine,* 2nd ed. Chevy Chase, MD: American Society of Addiction Medicine, 1998, p. 531.

41. Griffiths RR, Bigelow GE, Liebson IA: Human coffee drinking: reinforcing and physical dependence producing effects of caffeine. *Journal of Pharmacology and Experimental Therapeutics,* 1986; 239(2): 416–425.

42. Smith DE, Seymour RB: LSD: history and toxicity. *Psychiatric Annals,* 1994; 24(3): 145–47.

43. Schmitz JM, Henningfield JE, Jarvik ME: Pharmacologic therapies for nicotine dependence, in: Graham AW, Schultz TK, Wilford BB (eds.), *Principles of Addiction Medicine,* 2nd ed. Chevy Chase, MD: American Society of Addiction Medicine, 1998, p. 571.

44. Carroll KM: Characteristis of effective counselors, in: Graham AW, Schultz TK, Wilford BB (eds.), *Principles of Addiction Medicine,* 2nd ed. Chevy Chase, MD: American Society of Addiction Medicine, 1998, p. 609.

45. McLellan AT, Woody GE, Luborsky L, Goehl L: Is the counselor an "active ingredient" in substance abuse rehabilitation? An examination of treatment success among four counselors. *Journal of Nervous and Mental Disease,* 1988; 176: 423–430.

46. Miller WR, Benefield RG, Tonigan JS: Enhancing motivation for change in problem drinking: a controlled comparison of two therapist styles. *Journal of Consulting and Clinical Psychology,* 1993; 61: 455–461.

47. Prochaska JO: Enhancing motivation to change, in: Graham AW, Schultz TK, Wilford BB (eds.), *Principles of Addiction Medicine,* 2nd ed. Chevy Chase, MD: American Society of Addiction Medicine, 1998, p. 595.

48. Graham AW, Fleming MS: Brief interventions, in: Graham AW, Schultz TK, Wilford BB (eds.), *Principles of Addiction Medicine,* 2nd ed. Chevy Chase, MD: American Society of Addiction Medicine, 1998, p. 615.

49. Galanter M: Network therapy, in: Graham AW, Schultz TK, Wilford BB (eds.), *Principles of Addiction Medicine,* 2nd ed. Chevy Chase, MD: American Society of Addiction Medicine, 1998, p. 653.

50. Higgins ST, Tidey JW, Stitzer ML: Community reinforcement and contingency management interventions, in: Graham AW, Schultz TK, Wilford BB (eds.), *Principles of Addiction Medicine,* 2nd ed. Chevy Chase, MD: American Society of Addiction Medicine, 1998, p. 675.

7
Chapter Seven

Abstinence and Recovery:
The Clinician's Role

Treatment forms the bridge between active addiction and active recovery. It therefore behooves the health professional involved in providing treatment to have a working knowledge of what is involved in recovery so that he or she can help the addicted patient make the transition from treatment to recovery. Until relatively recently, there was very little connection or communication, or for that matter mutual understanding between the treatment and recovery communities. Once that connection began to be made, however, dramatic improvements in time clean and sober became apparent in patients who embraced a program of supported recovery. It also became increasingly apparent that those patients who were helped into recovery by understanding treatment personnel fared better than those who exited treatment and then sought out recovery on their own.

In the fall of 1990, Robert L. DuPont, M.D., director emeritus of both the President's Office for Substance Abuse Policy (OSAP) and the National Institute on Drug Abuse (NIDA) and John P. McGovern, M.D., Clinical Professor of Medicine at the University of Texas Medical School, Houston, convened an expert committee composed of individuals who were knowledgeable of 12-Step programs and/or social institutions, including health care, substance abuse treatment, education, religion, the workplace, and the criminal justice system. Topics at the 2-day meeting included the role of the 12-Step fellowships in treatment, accessibility to 12-Step meetings, appropriate introductory techniques, and the role of individuals and social institutions in the referral process. The result of the meetings was a book, *A Bridge to Recovery*,[1] which provides a detailed history of the recovery movement and descriptions of how a variety of institutions including health-care systems and substance abuse treatment facilities. The meetings provided a capstone to the recognition of recovery as a prime goal of addiction treatment and an acceptance of the health professional's role in furthering the transition.

It has become increasingly obvious that understanding the history and nature of recovery can be an important tool in the practitioner's repertoire, making it possible to initiate a patient's positive relationship with recovery even while treatment is in progress.

The 12-Step Movement and Its Fellowships

History tells us that the first 12-Step fellowship, Alcoholics Anonymous, was born in 1935 through an interaction between Bill W., a down-on-his-luck stock broker from New York, and Doctor Bob, a surgeon living in Akron, OH.[2] Both of these men came from white, middle-class backgrounds, as did most of the formative members of A.A., who helped to develop the steps and traditions that gave the fellowship and succeeding 12-Step fellowships their basic form and character. Their ideals and concepts for the new fellowship were rooted in the Oxford movement, a Christian fellowship that later became known as Moral Rearmament. When A.A. first became interrelated with treatment for alcoholics, it was through the Minnesota Model, developed at Hazelden with at least partial initial sponsorship from the Catholic Church.[3] The writing style found in the Big Book,[4] originally published in 1939, can also be seen to reflect the white, male, middle-class, Christian origins and values of its authors.

With such beginnings, one would expect there to be an ongoing adherence to Christianity and white middle-class values to the exclusion of other cultures within Alcoholics Anonymous and subsequent 12-Step fellowships. And yet, from its beginnings, elements within the "group conscience" of A.A. began working to broaden the scope and flexibility of their fellowship. Early on, the fellowship began to distance itself from the Oxford Movement, remaining friendly but moving toward a more eclectic spirituality that did not specify Christian dogma. In *Alcoholics Anonymous Comes of Age*[2] Bill W. speaks of how the 12 steps were re-phrased in their development to initiate such terms and concepts as "a higher power," and "God *as we understood him.*"

Alcoholics Anonymous may have had its specific beginnings in the Oxford Movement and the personal interaction between Bill W. and Doctor Bob, but its basic tenets reflect a spectrum of cultural antecedents, a number of which are discussed in *Drugfree: A Unique, Positive Approach to Staying Off Alcohol and Other Drugs.*[5] Throughout history and within various cultures, attempts have been made to deal with addiction and associated human problems. The most generally successful of these have involved in some way the development of individual spiritual maturity within a supportive environment. The authors see the 12 steps developed by Alcoholics Anonymous and adapted by other 12-Step fellowships as a blueprint for developing spiritual maturity, similar in intent to such entities as the Buddhist *Four Noble Truths* and *Eightfold Path*, the Hindu *Vedas*, and the Zen *Oxherding Panels*.

While the history of A.A. in the United States has been primarily one involving the European-American culture, the nature of the 12 steps and the precepts that underlie the fellowships can be seen as much more universal. This nature is both basic and flexible, lending itself to a wide range of interpretation and applications. In his book, *Physician, Heal Thyself!*, Dr. Earle M.[6] discusses his personal experiences with A.A. chapters in other cultures throughout the world. In his travels, Dr. Earle encountered Buddhist, Moslem and other A.A. chapters that had adapted A.A. to their own cultural needs and points of reference.

Individuals with certain religious backgrounds may have particular problems relating to certain tenets of the 12 steps. Many Buddhists, for example, venerate the Buddha as a fully enlightened being to be followed and emulated, but do not see him as a "higher power." These Buddhists, not utilizing a concept of God or a higher power in their cultural background, see their faith as a philosophy and a way of life rather than as a religion. Points of reference need to be established in order for 12-Step recovery to become meaningful for these individuals.

Narcotics Anonymous

The first Narcotics Anonymous (N.A.) meeting took place in Southern California in 1953. The new fellowship was started, with the help and encouragement of A.A. members, as an alternative to developing a special interest group within A.A. to be called "A.A. for Addicts." Growth of the fellowship was slow at first, but accelerated in the early 1980s with the publication of N.A.'s *Big Book*.[7] As of January,1988, there were over 12,000 N.A. meetings in over 43 countries. At that time, the fellowship was growing at a rate of 50% annually.[8]

This fellowship was started by addicts seeking recovery who felt that Alcoholics Anonymous, with its focus on the suffering alcoholic, did not fully meet their needs as individuals addicted to drugs other than alcohol. These individuals and the fellowship that followed, developed what they considered a broader spectrum program than that of A.A., through the recognition of other compulsive activities and self-destructive mechanisms as contributing factors in their addictions and through the acceptance of multiple addictions. Most young drug addicts today are addicted to more than one substance. In practice, a relative lack of slogans, an emphasis of formula-free personal communication, extended family orientation, and the custom of hugging one another in greeting, as well as N.A.'s attempts to stay aware of the changing drug milieu and treatment innovations, may make their program more appealing to young addicts.

In adapting the Twelve Steps to their needs, the only change made was the substitution of "addict" for "alcoholic" in the First and 12th Steps. This was done to show that N.A. dealt with the disease of addiction, not with any specific drug. In answer to the question, "Is N.A. only for narcotics addicts?" the N.A. answer is "No. We believe our problem is not the use of any specific drug or group of drugs. Our problem is the disease of addiction, and our program is one of abstinence from all drugs."[8]

Similarly, with the Twelve Traditions, the name Narcotics Anonymous was substituted for Alcoholics Anonymous and "drinking" was changed to "using" in the Third Tradition. For both documents, use and adaptation are by permission of A.A. World Services, Inc.

The Narcotics Anonymous Big Book[7] was published in 1982 and follows a concept and format somewhat similar to the A.A. Big Book. In it, one finds a Basic Text (pp. 1–101) that provides the long forms of the N.A. Steps and Traditions and general information on the principles of recovery from the disease of addiction. The second half, Book 2, is composed of "Personal Stories." Members of Narcotics Anonymous tell their stories, sharing their personal experiences, strength, and hope.

Narcotics Anonymous has a World Service Office, Inc., roughly analogous to Alcoholics Anonymous World Services, Inc., that is the publishing and distribution center for N.A. literature, and provides clerical and administrative services.[9]

Generally, N.A. meetings follow similar formats to their A.A. counterparts. Open meetings appear to be more structured than A.A.'s, and more oriented toward educating the visitor and potential newcomer about N.A.'s history, principles and operation.

Al-Anon and Alateen

Often, the relatives of the addicted patient are in need of support just as much if not more than the patient. For those individuals close to the patient, there are the fellowships of Al-Anon and Alateen. In its literature, Al-Anon Family Groups describes itself as a self-help fellowship offering a program of recovery for relatives and friends of alcoholics that is based on the Twelve Steps and Twelve Traditions as adapted from Alcoholics Anonymous. Alateen is referred to as a part of Al-Anon that is for younger family members who have been affected by someone else's drinking. The Twelve Steps and the Twelve Traditions are respectively the "heart" and "backbone," guarding the unity of the fellowship.

The Twelve Steps, as used by Al-Anon/Alateen, are nearly identical to those used by A.A.,[10] but there are several substantiative changes in the Twelve Traditions. Tradition Three, concerning individual membership in A.A.'s version, here includes group formation:

> 3. The relatives of alcoholics, when gathered together for mutual aid, may call themselves an Al-Anon Family Group, provided that, as a group, they have no other affiliation. The only requirement for membership is that there be a problem of alcoholism in a relative or friend.

The Fifth Tradition, regarding purpose, is also more detailed than the A.A. model:

> 5. Each Al-Anon Family Group has but one purpose: to help families of alcoholics. We do this by practicing the Twelve Steps of A.A. *ourselves* by encouraging and understanding our alcoholic relatives, and by welcoming and giving comfort to families of alcoholics.

Minor alterations are found in the Fourth Tradition, which alludes to the special relation between Al-Anon and A.A., and Eleventh Tradition, which adds: "We need guard with special care the anonymity of all AA members." Tradition Six makes clear the relationship between Al-Anon and A.A. by adding: "Although a separate entity, we should always cooperate with Alcoholics Anonymous."[11]

■ AL-ANON

Al-Anon began as a natural outgrowth of Alcoholics Anonymous called the Family Group. No one seems to know exactly when the first Family Group was started, but the precedent was apparently set by Anne and Lois, the wives of A.A. co-founders Dr. Bob and Bill W. and carried on by Katie, the wife of Earl T., who founded A.A.'s first Chicago group. Anne and Lois came early to the realization that many A.A. families needed the program just as much as their alcoholic members. They urged the Steps on non-alcoholic wives and husbands as a means of restoring normalcy to family life.[2]

The development of these Family Groups was based on the premise, only now gaining ground in the treatment community, that alcoholism/addiction is a family disease. Personal experience indicated that non-alcoholic family members were just as powerless over alcohol as their alcoholic parents, children, and spouses. Often, after the initial family-wide euphoria when the active alcoholic entered a program of abstinence and recovery, family members discovered that they were still on an emotional roller coaster. Wives and husbands either grew complacent and resentful of the time taken up by A.A. activities, or found that things continued to go badly at home. Sometimes conditions even got worse.

The Family Groups were based on the premise that change needed to take place in the non-alcoholic family members, and the conviction that a transformation could be brought about in their own lives by practicing the 12 steps in their own daily lives. As with the A.A. members, those in the Family Groups needed the company and support of other wives, husbands, parents, and children of alcoholics who were able to understand the problems faced by other members of alcoholic families. The message of these groups was that families could enjoy emotional as well as alcoholic sobriety. Further, even if the rest of the family hasn't found stability; even if the alcoholic hasn't achieved abstinence and recovery, the family member or members in a Family Group can have theirs and develop a personal emotional sobriety that will hasten the transformation of the rest of the family as well.

In 1954, Al-Anon incorporated as a separate world-wide fellowship known as Al-Anon Family Group Headquarters, Inc., and is no longer affiliated with A.A. or with any other organization.

Management of Al-Anon's World Service Office is guided by an annually elected voluntary Board of Trustees, an Executive Committee and a Policy Committee. In line with A.A. and N.A., it is self supporting and accepts no outside funding.

■ ALATEEN

Alateen is an outgrowth of Al-Anon that was established to provide young Al-Anon members, mostly teenagers, with their own forum in which to share experience, strength and hope with each other, discuss their difficulties, learn effective ways to cope with their problems, encourage one another, and help each other in understanding the principles of the Al-Anon program. Each Alateen group has a group sponsor who is an adult member of Al-Anon. The group sponsor's role is that of an active participant, who provides guidance and knowledge about the Steps and Traditions.

In Alateen, the members learn about the disease of alcoholism. Particularly, they become aware that, on the one hand, they are not the cause of anyone else's alcoholism or behavior, and on the other that they cannot change or control anyone but themselves. The program engenders the sense that despite alcohol-related family dysfunction, they can develop a satisfying and rewarding personal life. They can do this by recognizing and developing their own spiritual and intellectual resources. They can also continue to love the drinker or drinkers in their lives while detaching themselves emotionally from the drinker's problems. Aside from identifiers, the Steps and Traditions followed by Alateen are nearly identical to those of Al-Anon. Both fellowships share the same world headquarters.

Specialized 12-Step programs have proliferated in recent decades and now include Cocaine Anonymous, Marijuana Anonymous, Adult Children of Alcoholics, and Overeaters Anonymous. The more specialized groups are usually active in urban areas but may be hard to find in smaller towns and rural areas. In general, Alcoholics Anonymous has moved toward accepting a broader range of addictions, but this is not always the case. There are meetings that consider any addiction other than alcohol to be outside their scope. The referring physician or other therapist should become familiar with the nature of meetings in his or her area so as to make a compatible referral.

Non-Twelve-Step Recovery Programs

There are also a number of non-12-Step recovery programs, such as Rational Recovery, SMART Recovery, Secular Organizations for Sobriety (SOS), Men For Sobriety (MFS), and Women For Sobriety (WFS).

Rational Recovery was founded by Jack Trimpey, a social worker in 1986 and considers itself to be educational as opposed to therapeutic, eliciting a cure through rational thinking. The goal is disassociating the feelings that support use from those that support abstinence. Recovery is seen as an event rather than a process, one that represents a "cure" based on educational rather than therapeutic approaches.

SMART (Self-Management And Recovery Training) Recovery is a four-module program that purports to draw upon the latest scientific information on addiction. The motivational module involves motivating the addict to take action and get serious about sobriety. The DISARM (Destructive Self-talk Awareness and Refusal Method) module is designed to recall the negative experiences and consequences of drinking and other drug use and initiate behavioral "thought-stopping" through a variety of prompting devices to counter cravings. The REBT (Rational-Emotive Behavior Therapy) module works to defuse intense emotions before they inhibit rational thinking and provoke an urge to use. The first module deals with lifestyle changes, essentially filling the void left by abstinence and helping the addict find new people, hobbies, activities, and even career choices. Exercises involving relaxation and meditation training are employed to demonstrate enhancement of brain activity.

As the name implies, Moderation Management is about preventing alcohol abusers and problem drinkers from falling into addiction by providing information on alcohol, moderate drinking guidelines, drink monitoring exercises, goal-setting, and self-management within a context of developing moderation and balance in all aspects of life.

According to Gerstein,[12] most of these groups share the following elements:

- Permanent abstinence: With the exception of Moderation Management, all the rest advocate permanent abstinence as the goal of the treatment process.
- Recognition of the importance of choice in addiction care.
- Rejection of the "disease concept."
- Absence of labeling.
- Rejection of the concept of a lifetime in recovery.
- Acceptance of pharmacologic therapy.
- Unity of the addictions.
- De-emphasis on meeting frequency.
- Encouragement of discussion and crosstalk.

The Value of Alternative Recovery

The authors would add to the above the belief in secularization or de-spiritualization of the recovery process. While they feel that spirituality, as exemplified within the A.A. model 12-Step recovery fellowships is a key component to recovery and therefore continue to emphasize these fellowships, they also recognize the need for diversity in both treatment and recovery. In their 1989 review of alcoholism treatment literature, Hester and Miller[13] concluded the following:

- No single approach to treatment is superior for all individuals. In fact, different individuals respond to quite different treatment approaches.
- The state of the art is an array of empirically supported alcoholism treatment options.

- The appropriate question is not "Which treatments are best?" but "Which types of individuals are the most appropriate for a given program?"; "For this individual, which approach is most likely to succeed?"; "Is it possible to match individuals to optimal treatment, thereby increasing treatment effectiveness and efficiency?"

In essence, the same rules of diagnosis-driven treatment espoused by the American Society of Addiction Medicine apply to recovery. It is in the best interest of the patient to match him or her to the recovery fellowship or program that has the best chance of success with that particular patient.

Membership in 12-Step Fellowships

Generally speaking, there is no formal membership in a 12-Step fellowship. One does not fill out an application form. Beyond the passing of a voluntary donations container for such needs as coffee and meeting space rental, there are no dues, assessments, or membership fees. In fact, most groups do not keep membership records. Most individuals become associated with a fellowship simply by attending its meetings on a regular basis.

Just as there is no formal membership, or application procedure for a fellowship, there is no set membership for most specific meetings within a fellowship. Individuals are free to come and go, to attend this meeting or that meeting as frequently or infrequently as they see fit. While there may be a core of individuals who regularly attend a specific meeting, others come and go, attending different meetings depending on such factors as time, availability, individual preference, and need.

The fluidity of meetings can vary depending on group identity, location, and population density. In rural settings, where the fellowship population may be low and not very mobile, there may be little variation in meeting constituency. Urban and high-density suburban areas may offer a number of meetings available to a comparatively mobile fellowship population. In some instances, the constituency of a meeting and even its overall leitmotif may vary dramatically from week to week.

Meeting Structure

Twelve-Step meetings are typically held once a week, and may be 1–2 hours in duration. In Alcoholics Anonymous, they may have names that are more or less descriptive, such as "Monday Blues," "T.G. I'm Sober," etc. These meetings will often have a Secretary, an elected volunteer who convenes the meeting and assigns "commitments" to other volunteers in the group; a Treasurer, who takes responsibility for collecting the meeting donations and paying the bills; a representative to the local committee, who attends and reports on local committee meetings; and a refreshment person who makes coffee, tea, and provides appropriate refreshments at the meetings. The "coffee" person may set up the meeting, arranging or supervising the arrangement of chairs, etc., as necessary, or there may be a setup, and one or more cleanup volunteers. Larger meetings may have greeters and individuals designated to help "newcomers." All of these meeting functionaries are elected or appointed to fulfill these specific "commitments," usually for a period of 6 months. Meeting commitments are looked on as one means of developing and maintaining quality personal recovery, so there is usually no lack of volunteers.

A typical A.A. meeting will open with the secretary introducing him-or-herself as an alcoholic, welcoming everyone to the "Saturday Night Rap-Trap Meeting of Alcoholics Anonymous," often leading a recitation of "The Serenity Prayer," and asking one of the attendees to read "How It Works," from the "Big Book." "How It Works" contains the "12 Steps of Alcoholics Anonymous." Another attendee may be asked to read the "12 Traditions," either at this point or near the end of the meeting. The secretary may then ask newcomers and visitors from outside the area to introduce themselves by their first names only " ... so that we can get to know you and talk to you after the

meeting." Each such introduction is usually followed by supportive applause, and the secretary will officially welcome the newcomers and visitors.

Meetings often conclude with a reading of the "12 Traditions,"
perhaps a reading of the "Promises" (found on pp. 83–84 of the
Big Book) and a call for A.A.-related announcements. The meeting
ends with everyone standing, joining hands and observing a
moment of silence, and/or reciting "The Lord's Prayer," "The
Serenity Prayer," or whatever closing has been designated by the
meeting constituency as appropriate.

Meeting Types

Within this general structure, there are two specific meeting types.
Each of these has its own function within the fellowship. In general,
meetings are divided between open meetings and closed meetings.

■ OPEN MEETINGS

An open meeting is a group meeting that any member of the community can attend. It doesn't matter whether the person feels that
he or she is in need of the fellowship, or is a friend or loved one of
a member, or is merely curious. The only obligation placed on
attendance is that of honoring the anonymity of others by not dis-
closing their names outside the meeting. The views expressed at
these meetings are those of the individuals attending, in that all
A.A. members speak only for themselves. Open meetings usually
conclude with a social period at which coffee, soft drinks, cakes,
cookies, and other appropriate refreshments may be served.

■ CLOSED MEETINGS

In contrast, closed meetings are limited to members of the local fellowship group and visitors from other groups within the fellowship.

These meetings safeguard members anonymity and provide a forum for the discussion of specific phases of the members problems that may be understood best by fellow members of the specific fellowship. The meetings are usually informal and highly participatory. All members are encouraged to participate in discussions. Closed meetings can be particularly helpful for newcomers, especially those who may be concerned about their anonymity in the community. They also provide a forum for airing questions that may trouble a beginner, or even an old-timer, that may seem inappropriate for an open meeting but do merit serious discussion.

Groups composed of individuals with like interests, such as health professionals, may opt for a closed meeting format. This allows them to address specific issues that involve a professional interface within their fellowship that are important within the group but would not be appropriate to pursue in depth in an open meeting. For physicians, the closed format also provides a means of escaping the doctor/patient identity that can reassert itself if a patient or client is encountered at an open meeting.

Meeting Formats

Within the two types of 12-Step meetings, there are several primary meeting formats and a variety of sub-formats that meetings may adopt. These include the following.

■ DISCUSSION MEETINGS

Discussion meetings and speaker/discussion meetings are the two most common A.A. meetings, and similar formats are used by other 12-Step fellowships as well. In a discussion meeting, the secretary usually presides, either supplying a topic or asking if anyone in the group has a topic that they wish to discuss. Topics usually involve recovery and fellowship issues. They may vary considerably, although certain themes, such as exercising spirituality, dealing with fear, anxiety, and other personal recovery problems, interpersonal and other life problems, and dealing with the disease frequently recur. Anyone and everyone at the meeting is encouraged to speak, either on the topic or on their own particular concerns or issues. Each speaker, when recognized by the secretary, introduces him or herself by first name and fellowship designation, i.e., Jan, alcoholic; John, addict; Richard, junkie and drunk; Alice, a grateful alcoholic. The rest then say, "Hi Jan," or whoever, and the person says his or her piece. This process continues until the end of the meeting. In most meetings, "cross-talk," i.e., sustained dialogues between two individuals, is discouraged in the interest of making sure that the meeting time is not dominated by one or two members and that everyone who wants to can have their say.

■ SPEAKER AND SPEAKER/DISCUSSION MEETINGS

At a speaker or speaker/discussion meeting, a member of the fellowship is asked to speak at the meeting. In some situations, the speaker may occupy the center for the entire meeting, but in most cases it is understood that the speaker's story will be limited to half an hour. Speakers may be regular attenders at the meeting, or they may have never attended the meeting at which they are speaking. Secretaries often work for a balance of the familiar and the new. There is no rule to this effect, but it is generally thought that an individual should have at least 6 months in the fellowship before being a formal speaker.

The format most often used in a speaker's story can be expressed as, "what it was like, what happened, and what it is like now." In other words, the speakers are expected to talk about their life as dominated by addictive disease, how they came into the fellowship, and how their life has changed as a result of the fellowship. When they are done, the secretary will ask them to provide a topic for discussion, and the speaker acts as moderator for the rest of the meeting, which now has the same format as a discussion meeting.

The first time a member speaks at a meeting is an important personal occasion, a valedictory that marks a passage within the fellowship. Although speakers may find the experience difficult, it is nearly always a positive experience and an aid in strengthening one's program of recovery and sobriety.

■ STEP MEETINGS

The 12 Steps provide a blueprint for developing individual spiritual maturity with the fellowship, and as such have a special type of meeting all their own. These are the step meetings. When a step meeting is initiated, it usually starts work on Step 1 at its first session and continues to focus on a step at a time through number 12. Then it starts back on Step 1 again. Some meetings may work their way through the Twelve Traditions as well.

In A.A. step meetings, the meeting will usually start with passing around and reading aloud the appropriate step in its long form from the "Twelve by Twelve," *Twelve Steps and Twelve Traditions.*[14] The step, itself, then becomes the topic for discussion and the meeting follows a discussion format. A variation on this is a step/speaker meeting, in which the speaker is asked to organize the talk in relation to the step, and again, the step is the discussion topic.

■ BOOK MEETINGS

Book meetings are similar to step meetings but involve initiatory serial readings from the "Big Book," or other fellowship publications, such as *Living Sober: Some methods A.A. members have used for not drinking*[15] or *Came to Believe . . . : The spiritual adventure of A.A. as experienced by individual members.*[16] Once more, passages are read by those attending the meeting, and these provide the topic for discussion.

■ CHIP, OR BIRTHDAY MEETINGS

These are meetings at which fellowship birthdays are acknowledged. Members' birthdays are measured from their entry into the fellowship and are maintained as long as the member remains sober. Members who have a relapse typically admit this when they reenter the fellowship and set a new birth-date on their re-entry. Although a great deal of emphasis is placed on staying sober or drug-free "one day at a time," cumulative time in sobriety is encouraged and recognized through ceremonial recognition and the awarding of "chips," often literally poker chips that are engraved with the fellowship logo on one side and length of sobriety on the other. These are awarded by the meeting secretary or designee at the end of the meeting with general applause and encouragement. Chip meetings are usually open meetings and those close to a member receiving a chip are encouraged to attend.

Given the critical nature of early recovery, these tokens of accomplishment are given more frequently than the first year. Although there is no rule on this, the usual periods are: 24 hours, 30 days, 6 months, 1 year, and then at the end of each year thereafter. It is interesting to note that these intervals correspond with times that have been recognized as when the newly recovering individual is most vulnerable to relapse.

Frequent meetings other than chip meetings will set aside a few minutes at the last meeting of the month to recognize attendees who have birthdays in that month. Often special refreshments, such as a cake, are served as celebration of all members being a month older in sobriety.

Most often a meeting will adopt one format and use it every week. The meeting name may reflect the format, such as "Sunday Night Big Book Study," "Tuesday Night Step," "12 by 12 Study," or "Noon Discussion." Other meetings may vary their format, such as 3 weeks of speaker/discussion and once a month step study. There are no hard and fast rules on meeting format, and meetings vary to some extent between fellowships, regions, and groups.

Where Meetings are Held

Twelve-Step fellowship meetings may be held in just about any place that is available and will accommodate itself to the meeting needs. These may include churches and church meeting centers, school rooms, community centers, private homes, health centers, hospital wards, human service agencies, drug and alcohol treatment centers, cafeterias, and club rooms. In some areas, clubs have been established to accommodate fellowship members, providing an alcohol and other drug-free place for fellowship members to spend their time, and a center for meetings. The nonalcohol Alano Club, with its coffee bar, meeting and recreation rooms, is an example found in many parts of the United States.

Reading the 12-Step Fellowship Directory

Wherever 12-Step fellowship meetings exist, an information number for that fellowship will be listed in the local telephone book. When called, a volunteer will provide local meeting times, locations, and other pertinent information about local fellowship activities. These volunteers often have "on call" fellowship members who will respond to requests for help as part of their own 12th step work.

Many areas produce a regularly updated directory of local meetings that provide name, location, time, and other particulars. The entries may be listed by town, by time or by day, but a typical line entry may be something like the following:

PORTTOWN
Wed. 8:00 PM CI DI WHAT ITS LIKE NOW 222 Lake Dr. 2 mi.
w. of Porttown off I88, back room Lakeside Recreation Center.

Sets of initials following the time usually give added information about the meeting: if its a book, what book; open or closed; any special restrictions or qualifications. Here are some of the more common abbreviations used in directories:

5D Mon-Fri	BB Big Book	CC Childcare Available
6D Mon-Sat	Bg Beginners	Cl Closed
7D every day	Bk Book	Di Discussion

NS No Smoking	Sr Speaker	Wh Wheelchair Access
SD Spkr. & Disc.	SS Step Study	Wo Women
Sh Spanish	YP Young People	ST Steps/Traditions
Gy Gay	Ls Lesbian	Me Men

Alcoholics Anonymous also issues an annual International AA Directory that lists countries by geographical area: Africa; Asia & Indian Ocean Islands; Australia, New Zealand, Pacific Islands & Antarctica; Bermuda & Caribbean Islands; Europe; Mexico & Central America; Near & Middle East; and South America & Falkland Islands. General Service Offices, where they exist, are listed first, followed by Central/Intergroup Offices, groups, loners, and contacts by city.

Points of Resistance Among Health Professionals

Some cultures are heavily invested in treatment approaches to addiction that do not recognize recovery and its promises as the goal of addiction treatment. These treatment approaches may be based on the concept that addiction is not a disease but a cluster of symptoms and behaviors that are secondary to pre-existing psychopathology. In these terms, addiction is not a viable object for primary treatment, but rather something that will clear in the course of psychotherapy and recovery, therefore, is not a viable goal. Even though the efficacy of 12-Step recovery is generally recognized by addictionologists, the general treatment community in the United States is still somewhat divided on this issue. There are individual physicians and professors who will argue that the whole concept of addiction is an artifice, that drug and alcohol abuse in all its forms is a moral issue, to be dealt with primarily through the courts and the criminal justice system.

One way in which professional resistance is being countered in this country is through medical education. Providing medical students with first-hand knowledge of Alcoholics Anonymous and Narcotics Anonymous has been a goal at the University of Nevada since 1974, when substance abuse education was added to the medical curriculum. Today, this exposure includes attendance at one AA/NA meeting in the second year and four in the third year, with appropriate class work to meet educational objectives. These objectives include learning what happens at AA/NA meetings and becoming familiar with the importance of a home group, the role of sponsors, the pitfalls and benefits of working with the 12 steps, and the value of service, i.e., the recovering addict carrying the message to other suffering alcoholics and addicts. Students also learn the differences between spirituality and religion, the importance of the traditions, and the problems and paradoxes found in 12-Step fellowships. The goal of the program is to produce physicians with positive attitudes toward 12-Step fellowships and sufficient skills and knowledge to support clients in 12-Step programs.[17]

In France, where the Toxicomanes, or physicians dealing with chemical dependency, are heavily invested into a psychotherapeutic approach, there is professional denial that 12-Step programs exist, or if they do, are at all effective with French clients. Several toxicomanes maintained that even if they, themselves, championed 12-Step recovery and attempted to refer clients into recovery programs, the French, with their heritage of individual freedom and idiosyncratic behavior and belief, would never abridge their freedom by joining such fellowships as A.A. Health professionals in such wine-producing, and consuming countries as Italy, Spain, and France also expressed concern over the issue of addicts needing to maintain abstinence from all psychoactive substances. Wine, they maintained, is a food, and should not be included in such a blanket prohibition.

Acceptance of 12-Step recovery overseas has differed from culture to culture, from country to country, in some cases from community to community. In Scandinavia, for a studied example, some countries, such as Finland, Iceland, and Sweden have experienced phenomenal multiplication of existing A.A. groups over the past 20 years, while others, such as Denmark and Norway have experienced a decline in groups over the same period. With the advent of glasnost, narcologists in what is now the former Soviet Union discovered A.A. Since that time, treatment has been increasingly linked with recovery in Russia and other eastern European republics.[18,19]

The Importance of Spirituality in Meaningful Recovery......

Addiction medicine, and anyone treating alcoholics with a goal of abstinence and recovery cannot ignore spiritual issues, and the most important source of recovery-enhancing spiritual experience is found in participation in a 12-Step program. Qualities such as humility, inner strength, a sense of meaning and purpose, acceptance, tolerance, and harmony in one's life are all developed through the exercise of a spiritual program of recovery. In essence, spirituality is connectedness: to a higher power, to an inner strength, to the group. It is connectedness to that which is outside the limited personal identity that is the seat of the self-centered disease of addiction.

According to John Chappel,[20] the attainment of physical and mental health requires more than the belief that they can be experienced. Both require active effort and practice on the part of each individual. The specialist in addiction medicine or addiction psychiatry, and the non-specialist who is treating addicted patients, must have a working knowledge of the potential role of spirituality in enhancing recovery from addictions. Knowledge and skill in supporting a patient's spiritual experience and the work necessary to develop and maintain spiritual health do not require spiritual beliefs on the part of the health care professional. The atheist or agnostic physician is at no greater disadvantage than is the physician who smokes or is overweight in helping patients deal with those problems. In any case, it is important that the physician refrain from any attempt to persuade the patient to adopt a particular set of religious beliefs. In this context, the physician is offered the following guidelines, which have been adapted from principles articulated by the American Psychiatric Association:[21]

- Maintain respect for each patient's beliefs.
- Obtain information about the religious or ideologic orienta-tion and beliefs of patients so that they can be attended to in the course of treatment.
- If conflict arises in relation to such beliefs, handle it with a concern for the patient's vulnerability to the physician's attitudes.
- Develop empathy for the patient's sensibilities and parti-cular beliefs.
- Do not impose one's own religious, anti-religious, or ideo-logic concepts in the course of therapeutic practice.

Although powerful arguments can be made against including spiritual issues in addiction medicine, an even stronger case can be made for their inclusion. The experiences of so many recover-ing alcoholics and other drug addicts cannot be ignored. As physi-cians, it is useful for us to practice acceptance of the varied spiritual experiences of our patients and to support them as help-ing their recovery.[20]

Learning More About Addiction and Spirituality

A question at the core of this book is how can we, as professionals, learn more about the great range of what we need to know regard-ing addiction and spirituality. To the authors' minds, the best way to learn is to go forth. Some of the wise kings in history made a practice of traveling incognito among their subjects in order to get a true picture of conditions within their various domains. Similarly, in our own cultures, individuals seeking to learn more of their milieu have gained by engaging those who are on similar paths. Addiction professions need to learn all they can about both the process and the practice of recovery, and may accomplish that by engaging in a dialogue with the recovering community both at a conceptual level and by attending meetings. Similarly, interaction with church and civic groups can broaden the ability to both understand and work with the cultural and spiritual dynamics involved in the practice of recovery.

REFERENCES

1. DuPont RL, McGovern JP: *A Bridge to Recovery: An Introduction to 12-Step Programs.* Washington, DC: American Psychiatric Press, Inc., 1994.
2. Alcoholics Anonymous: *Alcoholics Anonymous Comes of Age: A Brief History of A.A.* New York: Alcoholics Anonymous World Services, 1957.
3. McElrath D: *Hazelden: A Spiritual Odyssey.* Center City, MN: Hazelden, 1987.
4. Alcoholics Anonymous: *Alcoholics Anonymous: The Story of How Many Thousands of Men and Women Have Recovered from Alcoholism.* 3rd ed. New York: Alcoholics Anonymous World Services, 1976.
5. Seymour RB, Smith DE: *Drugfree: A Unique, Positive Approach to Staying Off Alcohol and Other Drugs.* New York: Facts on File, 1987.
6. Earle M: *Physician Heal Thyself! 35 Years of Adventures in Sobriety by an AA "Old Timer."* Minneapolis, MN: CompCare, 1989.
7. Narcotics Anonymous: *Narcotics Anonymous.* Van Nuys: World Service Office, Inc., 1982.
8. Narcotics Anonymous: *A Guide to Public Information.* Van Nuys: World Service Office, Inc., 1989.
9. Narcotics Anonymous: *A Guide to Public Information.* Van Nuys: World Service Office, Inc., 1989.
10. Al-Anon: *Purpose & Suggestions.* New York: Al-Anon Family Group Headquarters, Inc., 1969.
11. Al-Anon: *Al-Anon is for Adult Children of Alcoholics.* New York: Al-Anon Family Group Headquarters, Inc., 1983.
12. Gerstein J: Rational recovery, SMART recovery and non-twelve step recovery programs, in: Graham AW, Schultz TK, Wilford BB (eds.), *Principles of Addiction Medicine*, 2nd ed. Chevy Chase, MD: American Society of Addiction Medicine, 1998, p. 719.
13. Hester RK, Miller WR: *Handbook of Alcoholism Treatment Approaches: Effective Alternatives.* New York, NY: Pergamon Press, 1989.

14. Alcoholics Anonymous: *Twelve Steps and Twelve Traditions.* New York: World Services, Inc., 1953.
15. Alcoholics Alcoholics: *Living Sober.* New York: World Services, Inc., 1975.
16. Alcoholics Anonymous: *Came to Believe...* New York: World Services, Inc., 1973
17. Chappel JN: Teaching medical students to use 12-step programs. *Substance Abuse,* 1990; 11: 143–150.
18. Buxton ME, Smith DE, Seymour RB: Spirituality and other points of resistance to the 12-step process. *Journal of Psychoactive Drugs,* 1987; 19(3): 275–286.
19. Smith DE, Buxton ME, Bilal R, Seymour RB: Cultural points of resistance to the 12-step recovery process. *Journal of Psychoactive Drugs,* 1993; 25(1): 97–108.
20. Chappel JN: Spiritual components of the recovery process, in: Graham AW, Schultz TK, Wilford BB (eds.), *Principles of Addiction Medicine,* 2nd ed. Chevy Chase, MD: American Society of Addiction Medicine, 1998, p. 725.
21. American Psychiatric Association: Committee on religion and psychiatry: guidelines regarding possible conflict between psychiatrists' religious commitments and psychiatric practice. *American Journal of Psychiatry,* 1990; 47: 542.

Chapter Eight

Common Medical and Psychiatric Complications of Abuse and Addiction

Drug abuse and addiction can produce a number of sequelae, as well as coexist with a variety of coexistent medical problems. In anticipating and dealing with these, the physician must be aware of the patient's general health and perform a careful medical evaluation, keeping in mind that complex, expensive, and even risky diagnostic evaluations are not a substitute for a thorough basic clinical evaluation. Writing in the American Society of Addiction Medicine manual, *Principles of Addiction Medicine,* Wartenberg points out that addiction can also be related to a number of physical ailments in both a causal and non-causal relation. These include ischemic heart disease, hypertension diabetes mellitus, various forms of cancer, sexually transmitted diseases, retroviral infections, hepatitis, tuberculosis, and a variety of infections that are associated with parenteral drug use.[1]

In discussing the parallel treatment of physical disorders, Wartenberg concludes: "Patients with addictive disorders may be seen in medical, surgical, obstetrical or psychiatric units or outpatient clinics, and may be under the care of physicians of different specialties. Only a minority receive care in dedicated units for treatment of addiction. The Addiction medicine specialist may be called upon to see the patient in consultation, or may be the attending physician. In whatever setting such patients are encountered, it is critical that they be afforded the same respect and dignity accorded to any patient. Health professionals often have very negative attitudes toward patients with addictive disorders, and this frequently leads to escalating negative behaviors on the part of both patient and staff. The addiction medicine specialist—whether physician, nurse, social worker, psychologist, or other dedicated health professional—thus must assist not only in the medical evaluation and management of the patient, but also in establishing firm behavioral contracts to assure that the mutual obligations of patient and staff are safely and effectively met. Improved attitudes, knowledge and skills on the part of caregivers can promote better care within the medical mainstream."

As treatment of patients with recognized addictive disease moves further into the mainstream, meeting these concerns becomes increasingly important. When the Haight Ashbury Free Clinics were founded in 1967, the concept of "non-judgmental treatment" became a cornerstone of the free clinic philosophy, considered important in light of prevailing physician and other health professional attitudes toward drug abusers. The concern continues and non-judgmental approaches are critical to the successful treatment of addicts.

Sequelae and Medical Problems Associated with Specific Drugs

While the cause and effect relationship between drug abuse and specific medical syndromes may not always be clear, and in some cases drug use may be an attempt to self-medicate existing medical problems, there are certain generalizations that can be made between specific drugs or drug groups and related medical problems. In general, the following medical problems, described on a drug-group by drug-group basis, may be a sign of abuse or addiction. The examining physician should use any and all as a heads up to look closely and question the patient's use of psychoactive substances, including alcohol and tobacco.

There are several good texts on medical problems; however the "Medical Disorders in the Addicted Patient" section of

ASAM's manual is the most up-to-date and complete reference for diagnosis and treatment. The following drug-by-drug synopsis is based on Wartenberg's chapter on Medical Syndromes Associated with Specific Drugs which appears in that section.[2]

■ ALCOHOL-RELATED PROBLEMS

Malnutrition

Alcoholics and other addicts entering treatment may present with malnutrition, a problem that will be dealt with in Chapter 12. They may require a formal nutritional assessment in some cases, however, height/weight ratio and serum albumen will be sufficient in most cases. Multivitamins and thiamin are generally a good addition during and after detoxification, while other supplements, such as niacin, pyridoxine, folic acid, and/or magnesium may be called for. Care should be taken in supplementing vitamin A, toxic in high doses, and calcium and vitamin D for possible hypercalcemia and calcium nephrolithiasis. Ideally, a dietitian/nutritionist should be part of the treatment team.

Neurological Problems

Neurological problems may include periods of memory loss, or blackouts during heavy drinking episodes. Wernicke-Korsakoff syndrome and dementia are common, but care should be taken to distinguish alcohol-induced dementia and such other causes as hypothyroidism, syphilis, vitamin B_{12} deficiency, lesions of the central nervous system (CNS), infections, or degenerative conditions. Other alcohol related problems may include alcoholic cerebellar degeneration, marchiafava-bignami disease and other degenerations of the corpus callosum, central pontine myelinolysis, and such neuropathies as tobacco–alcohol amblyopia (producing double vision and decreased acuity) sensory neuropathy (presenting with burning dysesthesias of the feet and hands), motor neuropathy (proximal weakness) and autonomic neuropathy (with orthostatic hypotension and possible gastric emptying abnormalities). The most common neurologic problems involve seizures, but prescribing drugs that reduce seizure threshold should be done with care. Underlying hypertension and coagulopathies may make hemorrhagic and thrombotic strokes more common in alcoholics.

Gastrointestinal System

Alcohol is particularly irritating to the gastrointestinal (GI) system and can produce stomatitis, esophagitis, gastritis and duodenitis, exacerbate and retard healing of peptic ulcers and promote the development of *Helicobacter pylori*. Patients presenting with dysphagia, early satiety, early morning abdominal pain, and/or anemia should be evaluated for alcoholism.

Hepatic Problems

The liver, which does much of the work in digesting alcohol, is highly vulnerable to acute fatty metamorphosis, alcoholic hepatitis, perivenular fibrosis, and cirrhosis. Enzyme studies should be repeated every 2 to 4 weeks with such patients.

Hematological Problems

Alcohol can produce a variety of anemias: microcytic from upper gastrointestinal blood loss and iron deficiency, macrocytic secondary to membrane defects, premature release of red cells from bone marrow, liver disease or folate deficiency, or normochromic secondary to marrow suppression and/or chronic disease. Mild thrombocytopenia is often seen in alcoholics and usually returns to normal within a week of abstinence.

Cardiovascular Problems

Alcohol ingestion can result in supraventricular arrhythmias, including paroxysmal atrial fibrillation or "holiday heart." Increased levels of catecholamines during withdrawal can precipitate supraventricular and ventricular arrhythmias. Long-term heavy drinking can result in congestive cardiomyopathy characterized by signs of congestion including insidious but progressive dyspnea, intolerance to exercise and edema. Chronic alcohol use is also associated with arterial hypertension, while withdrawal can significantly elevate blood pressure.

Endocrine, Metabolic, and Miscellaneous Problems

According to Wartenberg,[2] various endocrine and metabolic comorbidities can result from acute alcohol ingestion, which may produce pyertriglyceridemia, lipemic serum and in some, painful abdominal crises. Hyperuricemia resulting in gout and other sequelae may occur when alcohol interferes with urate excretion, while a myriad of metabolic imbalances including hypoglycemia, inhibited vasopressin levels and elevated release of corticotrophin may occur. Loss of magnesium through increased urination may reduce parathyroid hormone secretion and hypocalcemia, while loss of both magnesium and calcium can lead to muscle weakness, tetany, seizures, and cardiac arrhythmias. Production of male and female sex hormones can be reduced, resulting in impaired fertility, menstrual irregularities or amenorrhea in women and decreased spermatogenesis, infertility and erectile dysfunction in men. Miscellaneous problems related to alcohol addiction include aspiration pneumonia, nocturnal sleep apnea, long abscess, pulmonary tuberculosis, acute and chronic myopathy, rhadomyolysis, myoglobinuria, hypophosphatemia, osteoporosis with resulting fractures, and a number of cancers, including oropharyngeal, esophageal, gastric, pancreatic, hepatic, colon, and breast cancer.

■ OTHER SEDATIVE-HYPNOTIC DRUGS

While these drugs have similar effects to those of alcohol, they have not been identified with the scope of related medical problems that alcohol has. One property that can be considered a sequelae is the synchronistic effect these drugs may have when taken with alcohol or one another. Essentially, drugs such as the benzodiazepines which may be safe at relatively high dosages when taken on their own can become deadly when taken in combination with alcohol or other drugs in this group, producing respiratory depression, coma and death. This reaction has to do with variable rates of metabolization and how these effect blood-brain levels of different drugs. The liver is preferential in its digestion of certain chemicals, and given a choice between breaking down alcohol and a benzodiazepine it will concentrate on the alcohol, allowing the benzodiazepine to build up to a potentially fatal level in the brain.

Sedative hypnotics can produce cognitive impairments including amnesia, visual tracking, and reflex responses. Meprobamate overdose can cause a gelatinous bezoar in the gut that may require endoscopic removal, while glutethimide can produce marrow suppression and pancytopenia.

■ PROBLEMS WITH OPIOIDS

Aside from causing sedation and constipation, opioids are relatively non-toxic when used as prescribed. In abuse, non-cardiac pulmonary edema and heroin-induced nephropathy with glomerulonephritis leading to renal insufficiency, and various neurological syndromes including multifocal leukoencephalopathy and myelopathies may occur.

The *nor* metabolites of meperidine, propoxyphene and pentazocine can result in seizures, even at therapeutic levels. In the late 1970s, faulty synthesis of a street-preparation of meperidine introduced an industrial neurotoxic called MPPP. That contaminate directly attacked dopamine-producing cells in the substantia nigra area of users' brains, producing a Parkinson-like sequelae that paralyzed its victims. Parkinson medication provided some relief and paradoxically the cases and a study of the MPPP action provided much information on how Parkinson disease develops.

■ STIMULANT DRUGS

Cocaine and other stimulants, including amphetamine and methamphetamine are capable of producing serious and extensive organ toxicity. These drug produce extensive vasoconstriction and can produce profound acute vascular and cardiovascular problems: severe hypertension, cardiac arrhythmias, angina, myocardial infarction, and sudden death are seen as well as cerebrovascular accident with stroke. Seizures are common with cocaine injection or smoking and may be accompanied by acute hyperthermia, muscle rigidity, severe rhabdomyolysis myoglobinura, and renal failure. Metabolites produced by the combining of cocaine and alcohol may exacerbate these problems.

Chronic nasal insufflation of cocaine can produce ischemic necroses resulting in septum perforation, while smoking can result in reduced pulmonary diffusing capacity with hypoxia and dyspnea and potential pulmonary edema. Other problems can include pneumothorax and pneumomediastinum from vigorous inhalation, pulmonary infarction, alveolar hemorrhage, vascular thrombosis, ischemia of the GI tract and hepatic damage.

The main difference between cocaine and the amphetamines is that the latter has a longer half-life or effectiveness and may have correspondingly longer periods of complications.

■ TOBACCO

The smokable stimulant nicotine is in and of itself a systemic poison that can produce or exacerbate a full spectrum of pulmonary diseases including emphysema and lung cancer. It is also responsible for producing cancers of the mouth, esophagus, and other organs. It has also been implicated in a variety of heart ailments. Overall, it has been reported by a number of sources that tobacco is responsible for over 400,000 deaths annually in the United States alone.

■ MARIJUANA

The smoking of marijuana can produce a variety of respiratory and pulmonary sequelae. Older users may experience tachycardia and angina while increased head and neck cancers have been reported in some users. A number of other problems have been claimed for relation to gonadal dysfunction, immune suppression, and long-term psychiatric problems but such have not been proven.

■ HALLUCINOGENS

Similarly, medical problems resulting from hallucinogen use appear to be rare. LSD, mescaline, psilocybin, and psilocin may produce tachycardia and the possibility of cerebrovascular constriction. Evidence that MDMA and other psychedelic stimulants may be necrotic to serotonin receptor sites is still controversial. Several deaths have occurred that are related to idiosyncratic reactions to these drugs. The most problems have been seen with phencyclidine (PCP) which is often included with the hallucinogens. Besides severe psychotic reactions, PCP can cause hyperthermia, rhabdomyolysis, renal failure, and intractable seizures.

■ INHALANTS

The volatile substances that include organic solvents, anesthetic gases, nitrites, glues, refrigerants, and other industrial materials can produce extreme neurotoxicity up to and including permanent cognitive dysfunction and neuropathy. Propellant fluorocarbons can produce cardiac arrhythmias and sudden death. Paint thinner, gasoline, butane, etc., may produce pulmonary, hepatic, renal, and hematologic toxicity. Misuse of anesthetic gases can cause asphyxiation and arrhythmias. The nitrites can produce profound cyanosis and dyspnea as well as dangerously low blood pressure due to their vasorelaxant properties.

■ NEEDLE ABSCESSES AND OTHER SKIN-RELATED COMPLICATIONS

Some of the medical complications found in addicts are the result of needle use or of substances used to cut or bulk out drugs. Skin complications provide some of the most easily recognizable signs of injection drug abuse:

1. Needle-track scars are caused by unsterile techniques and the injection of fibrogenic particulate matter.

2. In addition, attempts to sterilize the needle by heating the tip with a match causes the deposit of carbon, which causes mild inflammatory reaction; subsequent repeated injection with such a needle causes tattooing or dark pigmentation at the point of entry of the needle. However, macrophages pick up the carbon, and the tracks become progressively lighter. Although most common on the arms, tracks can be found on almost any part of the body, because abusers realize that the arms are the first area to be checked. Even the penile veins have been used for injection. The subcutaneous scars found on the thighs and arms are due to chronic abscesses.

3. Abscess formation (the most common septic problem) is usually easy to recognize. Repeated injections without cleansing the skin around the injection sites produce infections that are most commonly due to skin flora such as *staphylococci* and *streptococci*. Anaerobic infections, however, occur at a much higher rate in the drug user who injects. These abscesses may sometimes be recognized by the presence of a foul-smelling discharge, less often by gas formation, and by a bizarre type of cellulitis.

4. This cellulitis is characterized by a stony or wooden-hard tenseness, which progresses rapidly on an extremity, and not necessarily in association with a recent needle puncture or an infected site. Cellulitis occurs when sedative-hypnotics are injected subcutaneously. The tissue becomes reddened, hot, painful, and swollen.

5. Another complication in an extremity may be caused by intraarterial injection. Intense pain is usually produced distal to the site of injection. Swelling, cyanosis, and coldness of the extremity indicate the onset of a medical emergency. If this condition is untreated, gangrene of the hands or fingers may develop with consequent loss of these parts.

6. Campodactyly or permanent flexion of the fingers can result from recurrent use of the hand veins for injection. Irreversible contracture of the fingers and lymphedema may result.[3,4]

■ COMMUNICABLE DISEASES SPREAD BY NEEDLE USE AND UNSAFE SEX

In recent years the spread of major and often fatal disease through shared and otherwise contaminated needles has become a major health concern. HIV and AIDS are only the tip of the iceberg that includes the but recently identified hepatitis C virus that infects increasing numbers of even short-term needle users. Drug use can also cloud the judgment of individuals who engage in unsafe sexual practices, often with multiple partners. Prevention efforts involving frank discussions of needle hygiene and use of condoms and other protective devices is called for, particularly with teens.

Dual Diagnosis: Combined Addiction and Psychiatric Problems

A growing number of chemically dependent individuals, over 40% at the Haight Ashbury Free Clinics drug treatment sites, are under treatment for the condition known as "dual diagnosis." This is usually defined as a person having both a substance abuse problem and a diagnosable, significant psychiatric problem.

The psychiatric disorders most often seen in dual diagnosis in combination with drug abuse are

- major depression,
- schizophrenia (thought disorder),
- bipolar disorder (manic-depression).

Many treatment professionals also include other mental problems in their definition of dual diagnosis. These include:

- anxiety disorders, e.g., panic disorders, obsessive–compulsive disorders, post-traumatic stress syndromes,
- organic disorders,
- attention deficit/hyperactivity disorder (AD/HD),
- developmental disorders,
- somatoform disorders,

- rage disorders,
- other disorders, such as sexual dysfunction and anorexia.

A cocaine user might also have a psychosis or paranoia even when not using drugs. An alcoholic might have severe depression which persists even when the user is clean and sober. However, not every addict who exhibits psychotoform symptoms is a victim of dual diagnosis. It is important to distinguish between having symptoms and having a major psychiatric disorder. Everyone feels blue and sad sometimes. Everyone has the capacity for grief and loneliness, but this does not mean that a person is medically depressed, requiring medication or psychiatric treatment. It is really a question of severity and persistence of these symptoms.

■ FOUR PATTERNS OF DUAL DIAGNOSIS

Psychoactive substances can be related to four different patterns of dually diagnosed patients.

Pre-existing Mental Illness

One kind of dual diagnosis involves the person who has a clearly defined mental illness and then gets involved in drugs, for example the teen with major depression who discovers amphetamines.

Potential Mental Illness

Another kind of dual diagnosis associated with the use of psychoactive drugs occurs when there might be an underlying psychiatric problem that is not fully developed as yet. There is no clear-cut depression nor clear-cut schizophrenia before drug use begins. There may be some unusual thought patterns but these are not significant enough to be recognized as a mental illness. When that person starts to use psychoactive drugs, the effects of those substances activate or accelerate the development of the underlying mental disturbance.

Permanent, Drug-Induced Mental Illness

The third kind of dual diagnosis happens when there is not a pre-existing problem, but as a result of years of use or some extreme reaction to the drug, the user develops a chronic psychiatric problem because the toxic effects of the drug permanently imbalance the brain chemistry.

"Temporary," Drug-Induced Mental Illness

There is a fourth condition that is not really dual diagnosis which occurs when the drug itself or withdrawal from the drug causes a transient depression, temporary psychosis, or other apparent mental illness. The imbalance in the brain chemistry in this type of diagnosis is usually temporary, and with abstinence, the mental illness will disappear within a few months to a year. This is not true dual diagnosis but only a temporary condition resulting from the toxic emotional effects of the drug.[5]

■ DIAGNOSIS AND ASSESSMENT

When people see a relative or friend acting oddly and having trouble coping with everyday life over a prolonged period, they do not know whether they should ascribe it to relationship problems, trouble at home, drug use, or mental illness. Substance abuse and mental health professionals have the same problem. Thus, when assessing mental illness in a substance abuser, a general rule used by both mental health and substance abuse treatment professionals is that the initial diagnosis should be tentative, or as one psychiatrist said, *"The diagnosis should be written in disappearing ink because as the drug clears, the symptoms will change."*[6]

The prevalence of dual diagnosis depends on when the diagnosis is made. Since many mental symptoms are a temporary result of drug toxicity or drug withdrawal, an early diagnosis may merely be drug toxicity rather than dual diagnosis. Thus, the prudent chemical dependency clinician treats all dangerous symptoms but holds off making a psychiatric diagnosis until the drug user has had time to get sober and out of a state of drug intoxication or drug withdrawal.

- a reliance on prescribed medications such as antidepressants or antipsychotics so more clients are treated on an outpatient basis;
- increased reliance, in general, on outpatient mental health facilities.

Outpatient mental health clients are more likely to exhibit poor control of their prescribed medication thus aggravating their mental problems and making them more likely to turn to street drugs for help. Many people with mental disorders self-medicate with alcohol, heroin, amphetamines, or other drugs in an attempt to control their symptoms. As a result, the incidence of dual diagnosis among compulsive drugs users and particularly among the homeless remains extremely high.[7]

The growth of licensed professionals working in the field of chemical dependency treatment has resulted in a greater recognition and documentation of dual diagnosis. Increased abuse of cocaine and amphetamines has also increased the problem of dual diagnosis. A larger number of substance abusers means that more of them will also be dually diagnosed. Also, since stimulants are more toxic to brain chemistry than most substances, those with fragile brain chemistry are more likely to be pushed over the edge into chronic neurochemical imbalance and mental illness.[8]

In the past, inability to treat a person who manifested both a drug and a mental problem, combined with an outright refusal to develop treatment strategies for the dually diagnosed client, resulted in inappropriate and potentially dangerous interactions with clients. They were often shuffled aimlessly back and forth between the mental health-care system and the chemical dependency system without receiving adequate treatment. Even though there has been an increase in facilities that address the dually diagnosed client, inappropriate care is all too often still the rule rather than the exception.

Treating the Dual Diagnosed Patient

The dual diagnosed patient must be treated for both disorders and is best treated in a single program when appropriate resources are available. Where programs equipped to handle dual diagnosis (DD) cases are not available, CD programs need to establish linkages with mental health service providers and vice versa, so that they can work together in providing the client with their combined treatment expertise. Each needs to recognize that mental health and substance abuse treatment are both long-term propositions and, therefore, they need to establish both short-term and long-range services to address the problems of dual diagnosis.[9]

Multiple Diagnoses

As the chemical dependency treatment community becomes more aware of other simultaneous disorders which complicate the treatment of addiction, it must be willing to accept new challenges, such as:

- multiple drug (polydrug) addiction;
- chronic pain in the chemically dependent individual;
- other medical disorders such as epilepsy, cancer, heart and kidney disease, diabetes, sickle cell anemia, and even sexual dysfunction.

In addition, a variety of medical disabilities, such as hearing impairment and mobility impairment, and social concerns, such as cultural attitudes toward chemical dependency and mental health treatment and language barriers, may also provide impediments to successful treatment.

These problems require the development of future drug programs that are holistic, use several modalities, and are multidisciplinary in order to meet the challenge of the evolving, complicated, clinical needs of the chemically dependent patient.

■ MENTAL DISORDERS MOST OFTEN ASSOCIATED WITH SUBSTANCE ABUSE

Schizophrenia

Schizophrenia is a thought disorder believed to be mostly inherited, characterized by

- hallucinations (false visual, auditory, or tactile sensations and perceptions);
- delusions (false beliefs);
- an inappropriate affect (an illogical emotional response to any situation);
- autistic symptoms (a pronounced detachment from reality);
- ambivalence (difficulty in making even the simplest decisions);
- poor association (difficulty in connecting thoughts and ideas);
- poor job performance;
- strained social relations;
- an impaired ability to care for oneself.

The signs have to be present for at least 6 months for the diagnosis to be made.

Several abused drugs mimic schizophrenia and psychosis, producing symptoms which can be easily misdiagnosed. Cocaine and amphetamines, especially when used to excess, will cause a toxic psychosis that is almost indistinguishable from a true paranoid psychosis. Steroids can also cause a psychosis. Drug-induced paranoia can be indistinguishable from true paranoia. Most drugs, but particularly the uppers, MDMA ("ecstasy") and related stimulant/hallucinogens, and even marijuana, can cause paranoia.

The psychedelics, such as LSD, peyote, and psilocybin, and the multireaction drug PCP disassociate users from their surroundings, so all hallucinogen abuse can also be mistaken for a thought disorder. Also, withdrawal from downers can be mistaken for a thought disorder because of extreme agitation. Many of the psychiatric symptoms should disappear as the body's drug levels subside upon treatment and detoxification.

Major Depression

Major depression is classified as an affective disorder along with bipolar affective disorder and dysthymia (mild depression). A major depression is likely to be experienced by 1 in 20 Americans during their lifetime. It is characterized by

- depressed mood;
- diminished interest and diminished pleasure in most activities;
- disturbances of sleep patterns and appetite;
- decreased ability to concentrate;
- feelings of worthlessness;
- suicidal thoughts.

All of these symptoms may persist without any life situation to provoke them. For example, a patient with major depression may win a lot of money in a lottery and respond to it by being melancholy or depressed.

For the diagnosis to be made accurately, these feelings have to occur every day, most of the day for at least 2 weeks running. Organic causes, such as an illness or drug abuse, should rule out a diagnosis of major depression, as should natural reactions to the death of a loved one, separation, or a strained relationship.

The withdrawal symptoms which occur with most stimulant addictions (cocaine or amphetamine) and the come down or resolution phase of a psychedelic (LSD, "ecstasy") result in temporary drug-induced depression which is almost indistinguishable from that of major depression.

Bipolar Affective Disorder (Manic Depression)

This illness is characterized by alternating periods of depression, normalcy, and mania. The depression phase is described above. The depression is as severe as any depression seen in psychiatry. If untreated, many bipolar patients frequently attempt suicide. The mania, on the other hand, is characterized by

- a persistently elevated, expansive, and irritated mood;
- inflated self-esteem or grandiosity;
- decreased need for sleep;
- more talkative than usual or pressure to keep talking;
- flight of ideas;
- distractibility;
- increase in goal-directed activity or psychomotor agitation;
- excessive involvement in pleasurable activities that have a high potential for painful consequences (e.g., drug abuse, gambling, or inappropriate sexual advances). These mood disturbances are severe enough to cause marked impairment in job, social activities, and relationships.

Bipolar affective disorders usually begins in a person in their 20s and affects men and women equally. Many researchers believe this disease is genetic. Toxic effects of stimulants or psychedelic abuse will often resemble a bipolar disorder. Users experience swings from mania to depression depending upon the phase of the drug's action, the surroundings, and their own subconscious feelings and beliefs.

Anxiety Disorders

Anxiety disorders are the most common psychiatric disturbances seen in medical offices. There are

1. Panic disorder with and without agoraphobia (fear of open spaces).
2. Agoraphobia without history of panic disorder (a generalized fear of open spaces).
3. Social phobia (fear of being seen by others to act in a humiliating or embarrassing way, such as eating in public).
4. Simple phobia (irrational fear of a specific thing or place).
5. Obsessive-compulsive disorder (uncontrollable, intrusive thoughts and irresistible, often distressing actions, such as cutting one's hair or repeated hand washing).
6. Post-traumatic stress disorder (persistent reexperiencing of the full memory of a stressful event outside usual human

experience, e.g., combat, molestation, car crash). It is usually triggered by an environmental stimulus, i.e., a car backfires and the combat veteran's mind relives the stress and memory of combat. This disorder can last a lifetime and be very disabling.

7. Generalized anxiety disorder (unrealistic worry about several life situations that lasts for 6 months or more).

Sometimes it is extremely difficult to differentiate the anxiety disorders. Many are defined more by symptoms than specific names. Some of the more common symptoms in anxiety disorders are shortness of breath, muscle tension, restlessness, stomach irritation, sweating, palpitations, restlessness, hypervigilance, difficulty in concentrating, and excessive worry. Often anxiety and depression are mixed together. Some physicians think that many anxiety disorders are really an outgrowth of depression.

Toxic effects of stimulant drugs and withdrawal from opioids, sedatives, and alcohol (downers) also cause symptoms similar to those described in anxiety disorders and can be easily misdiagnosed as such.

Organic Mental Disorders

These are problems of brain dysfunction brought on by physical changes in the brain caused by aging, miscellaneous diseases, injury to the brain, or psychoactive drug toxicities. Alzheimer's disease, where older people suffer unusual rapid death of brain cells resulting in memory loss, confusion, and loss of emotions so they gradually lose the ability to care for themselves, is one example of an organic mental disorder. Mental confusion from heavy marijuana use in an elderly patient may mimic symptoms of this disorder.

Developmental Disorders

These include mental retardation, eating disorders, gender identity disorders, attention deficit disorders, autism, speech disorders, and disruptive behavior disorders. Heavy and frequent use of psychedelics like LSD or PCP can be mistaken for developmental disorders.

Somatoform Disorders

These disorders have physical symptoms without a known or discoverable physical cause and are likely to be psychologically caused, e.g., hypochondria (abnormal anxiety over one's health accompanied by imaginary symptoms of illness). Cocaine, amphetamine, and stimulant psychosis create a delusion that the users skin is infested with bugs when no infection exists.

The Passive-Aggressive, Antisocial, and Borderline Personality Disorders

These disorders are characterized by inflexible behavioral patterns that lead to substantial distress or functional impairment. Most of these personalities act out, that is, exhibit behavioral patterns that have an angry, hostile tone, that violate social conventions, and that result in negative consequences. Anger is intrinsic to all three of these personality disorders, as are chronic feelings of unhappiness and alienation from others, conflicts with authority, and family discord. These disorders frequently coexist with substance abuse and are particularly hard to treat because of the acting out, which is usually relapsing to drug use or creating a major disruption in their treatment.

Psychoanalysis and psychotherapy help clients explore their past to enable them to neutralize or minimize the emotional and neurochemical imbalance caused by heredity or the traumas and stresses of childhood, e.g., remembering sexual abuse that happened when they were young.

Individual or group therapy can be effective but, by necessity, it has to be a long-term undertaking (even a lifetime project) to be truly effective in changing individuals or at least in minimizing the damage they do to themselves.

■ PSYCHOACTIVE DRUGS AND TREATMENT

Psychoactive drugs themselves can be used to treat mental illness. This form of treatment is attempted by both psychiatrists and by patients themselves who may self-medicate their condition with the use of abusable drugs. Of course, there are dangers in self-medication. The uncontrolled use of street drugs, such as cocaine or some prescription medications like Ritalin®, can distort one's neurochemistry and thereby magnify or trigger mental problems.

Psychotropic medications (e.g., antidepressants, antipsychotics or neuroleptics, anti-anxiety drugs) that are prescribed by physicians to try to counteract neurochemical imbalance caused by mental illness or addiction can help the dually diagnosed client to lead a less destructive life.

■ DEVELOPMENTAL ARREST

Drug abuse and mental illness often result in a pause in emotional development. Take the case of a young man in his late teens or early 20s who is full grown and intelligent, but has been using drugs since the age of 11 or 12 and has also had emotional and mental problems. This type of patient comes to treatment with all kinds of difficulties. One of the worst problems is that he has suffered developmental arrest at age 11 or 12, the point where most people begin to work through issues and stresses in their lives. Most people mature through all the struggles and go on to become adults, but those who use drugs, who have avoided difficult emotions, and have not gone through that process of maturation will still experience the emotions that they avoided 5 or 6 years ago.

■ MEDICATING PSYCHIATRIC ILLNESS

Quite often, the dual diagnosis patient does need medication for the psychiatric disorder: tricyclic antidepressants for endogenous depression, lithium for a bipolar disorder (e.g., manic depression), and antipsychotic (neuroleptic) medication for a thought disorder. These medications have to be handled carefully because the individual has difficulty dealing with drugs. The clinician has to make sure that the medication used for the psychiatric problem does not aggravate or complicate the substance abuse problem.

Medications are used on a short-term, medium-term, or even lifetime basis to try to rebalance the brain chemistry that has become unbalanced either through hereditary anomalies, environmental stress, and/or the use of psychoactive drugs. They are used in conjunction with individual or group therapy and with lifestyle changes.

One of the biggest debates in treatment centers is about the level of medication that should be used. Some clinicians look at psychotropic medications as a last resort. Others feel that they should be the first step in treatment. However, there is no question that judicious use of many medications has freed many people suffering from mental illness from a life of misery.

■ PSYCHIATRIC MEDICATIONS AND THE RECOVERING COMMUNITY

One of the advantages of physician-prescribed medications over street drugs is that generally, except for the benzodiazepines and stimulants, they are not addicting. But sometimes, prescribing psychiatric medications for clients can cause problems for dually diagnosed clients because they are often taught to stay away from all drugs during recovery.

When using street drugs, patients feel a great deal of control over which drugs they ingest, inject, or otherwise self-administer. The same patients, when receiving medication from a doctor, often express the feeling that they are not in control any more of what is being given to them. Thus, they are more apt to rely on street drugs rather than on psychiatric medications for relief of their emotional problems.

■ VARIETIES OF PSYCHIATRIC MEDICATION

Some of the major groups of psychotropic medications are tricyclic antidepressants, MAO inhibitors, serotonin reuptake inhibitors, antipsychotics (neuroleptics), anxiolytics (anti-anxiety drugs), lithium, beta blockers, and sleeping pills.

Treating Depression

Many in the psychiatric field feel that depression causes and in turn is caused by an abnormality of the neurotransmitters norepinephrine (adrenaline) and serotonin, plus a few other neurotransmitters. Antidepressants are meant to increase the amount of serotonin or norepinephrine available to the brain to correct this imbalance.

Tricyclic Antidepressants

Tricyclic antidepressants such as imipramine (Tofranil) and desipramine (Norpramine) are thought to block reabsorption of these neurotransmitters by the sending neuron and so increase the activity of those biochemicals. This blocking effect, in turn, forces the synthesis of more receptor sites for these neurochemicals. The delay in the creation of new receptor sites may account for the lag time in effecting a change in the patient's mood. It usually takes 2–6 weeks for a patient to respond to the drug.

The tricyclics are very effective on patients with chronic symptoms of depression. People without depression do not get a lift from tricyclic antidepressants as they do with a stimulant. In fact, most of these medications actually cause drowsiness.

The tricyclic antidepressants, available mainly as pills, can be dangerous if too many are taken, so careful monitoring of not only compliance by the patient with prescribed dosage but also constant feedback from the patient as to the effects and side effects are also necessary. Major side effects are dry mouth, blurred vision, inhibited urination, hypotension, and sleepiness.

These drugs are also dangerous to the heart, especially if they are taken with stimulants, depressants, or alcohol. Patients must abstain from abusing drugs while being treated with tricyclic antidepressants.

Monamine Oxidase Inhibitors

MAO inhibitors such as phenelzine (Nardil), tranylcypromine (Parnate), and isocarboxazid (Marplan) are also used to treat depression. These very strong drugs work by blocking an enzyme which metabolizes neurotransmitters including norepinephrine and serotonin. This, in essence, raises the level of these neurotransmitters. Unfortunately, MAO inhibitors have several potentially dangerous side effects, so care and close monitoring are necessary in their use. They do give fairly quick relief from a major depression and panic disorder, but the user has to be on a special diet and remain aware of the possibility of high blood pressure, headaches, and several other side effects. Combined use of MAO inhibitors with abused stimulants, depressants, and alcohol can be fatal.

Newer Antidepressants

The newer antidepressants such as Prozac, Deseryl, Paxil, Zoloft, Welbutrin, and Xanax work through a variety of mechanisms.

Prozac® *(fluoxetine).* The most popular of the new anti-depressants, Prozac has received a large amount of publicity both pro and con since its release in 1988. It seems quite effective in the treatment of depression with fewer side effects than tricyclic antidepressants or the MAO inhibitors. It is also used to treat obsessive–compulsive disorders and panic disorder.

Prozac is classified as a serotonin reuptake inhibitor because it increases the amount of serotonin available to the nervous system. The amount needed to be effective varies widely from patient to patient and has to be adjusted. It generally takes 2–4 weeks for the full effect to be felt. The side effects are usually insomnia, nausea, diarrhea, headache, and nervousness. Most of the side effects are mild and will disappear in a few weeks.

Paroxetine (Paxil) and sertraline (Zoloft) also work to block serotonin uptake and have similar side effects as Prozac.

Xanax. Alprazolam (Xanax®), a benziodiazepine sedative-hypnotic, though not labeled as a treatment for depression, has been used clinically by several doctors to control mild depression or mixed depression and anxiety, but if the patient also has a drug problem, benzodiazepines are only recommended for detoxification or immediate relief.

Stimulants

In the past, amphetamine or amphetamine congeners such as Dexedrine, Biphetamine, Desoxyn, Ritalin, and Cylert were used to treat depression. They work by increasing the amount of norepinephrine and epinephrine in the CNS. They were mood elevators when used in moderation, but the problem was that since tolerance develops rapidly, and the mood lift proved to be too alluring, misuse and addiction developed fairly rapidly with the drugs. The overuse led to various physical and mental problems such as agitation, aggression, paranoia, and psychosis. Ritalin is occasionally prescribed for elderly patients with depression and for young patients with attention deficit disorder. But for a dually diagnosed client, these drugs should be used with utmost caution.

■ DRUGS USED TO TREAT BIPOLAR DISORDER (MANIC DEPRESSION)

Antidepressants such as the tricyclics or, recently, Welbutrin (bupropion) or Prozac, are initially used to treat severe depression in the bipolar patient and antipsychotics such as Thorazine or Haldol are initially used to treat the severe manic phase, but the main drug used for the treatment of bipolar illnesses over the last 30 years is lithium.

Lithium

Lithium is started concurrently with an antidepressant or an antipsychotic. Lithium is a long-term medication taken for years, even a lifetime. Clinicians are careful when making the diagnosis since the patient might be in the manic phase which resembles schizophrenia or the depressive phase which resembles unipolar depression. Misdiagnosis can be dangerous since long-term treatment of these other conditions is quite different.

Lithium does not really prevent a person from having moods. The patients still have high and low swings. What it does is dampen them. Because the high swings are not as high and the depressions are not as low, lithium helps the bipolar patient to function. About 80% of bipolar patients respond to lithium. Symptoms begin to change within 10–15 days after starting the drug.

Tegretol (carbamazepine) is used in patients who do not respond to lithium alone. It seems to help patients who have more rapid "cycling" of their highs and lows.

Depakene (valproic acid) is used if the bipolar patient fails to respond to lithium and Tegretol. Its use with the bipolar patient is still limited to cases resistant to other medications.

■ DRUGS USED TO TREAT SCHIZOPHRENIA (ANTIPSYCHOTICS OR NEUROLEPTICS)

In the early 1950s, a new class of drugs, phenothiazines, were found to be effective in controlling the symptoms of schizophrenia. Some of the drugs such as Thorazine, Mellaril Proloxin, and Compazine were initially referred to as major tranquilizers. More recently, non-phenothiazines like Haldol, Loxitane, and Moban have been developed. They act like phenothiazines and have similar side effects.

Researchers found that one of the major causes of schizophrenia is an excess of dopamine, a condition that is usually inherited. Most of the antipsychotic medications work by blockading the dopamine receptors in the brain, thereby inhibiting the effects of the excess dopamine. Generally, antipsychotic drugs do work, but they do not cure schizophrenia. They can also cause serious side effects. The difference in side effects is the main difference between many of the drugs.

The main side effects of antipsychotics usually have to do with the decrease in dopamine in the system. Dopamine controls muscle tone and motor behavior. By decreasing the dopamine, symptoms such as ticks, jumpiness, and inability to sit still are common. Parkinsonian syndrome (mainly a tremor but also loss of facial expression and slowed movements), akathisia (agitation, jumpiness—exhibited by 75 percent of patients), akinesia (temporary loss of movement and apathy), and even the more serious tardive dyskenesia (involuntary movements of the jaws, head, neck, trunk, and extremities) are the most common complications when using these medications. Often, a drug is given to block side effects, drugs such as Cogentin, Artane, or Kemadrin, or even Benadryl.

Patients on antipsychotics can seem drugged, but for people suffering from schizophrenia who are agitated or violent, the sedative effect is very useful. These drugs are dangerous when used as a sleeping pill by patients who do not have schizophrenia or are not violent and agitated. The drugs can actually cause symptoms of mental illness in patients who are not schizophrenic. They also have severe side effects.

Antipsychotic drugs in general are also classified as high potency (Haldol®, Stelazine®, Prolixin, Trilafon, Navane), and low potency (Thorazine Mellaril, Loxitrane, Moban).

In an emergency situation, patients are generally started on a high-potency antipsychotic. They are given several weeks to obtain a full response. If there is no response, either the dose can be raised or another drug tried. Most clinicians prefer to use low doses of these medications. The low-potency antipsychotics are used when patients also have problems sleeping. Manic patients are candidates for low-potency antipsychotic use.

Since antipsychotics are so potent, attempts are made to stop or decrease the dose of these medications as soon as possible, i.e., when the symptoms subside. This philosophy is particularly important in treating elderly patients.

Recently, atypical antipsychotic drugs have been tested. Clozaril (clozapine) is effective in the 30 percent of patients who do not respond to standard antipsychotic drug therapy. Unfortunately, weekly blood tests are necessary to monitor the side effects of Clozaril which make its use very expensive.

Patients who have been dually diagnosed with schizophrenia often self-medicate with heroin and other opioids to control their symptoms. Alcohol, other sedative-hypnotics, and even marijuana or inhalants are used as well. Since all of these street drugs have dangerous toxic effects when combined with antipsychotic drugs, patients are exhorted to cease using them while under psychiatric treatment.

■ DRUGS USED FOR ANXIETY DISORDERS

For generalized anxiety disorder, as well as some of the other anxiety disorders, the benzodiazepines are widely used. The most commonly used are Xanax, Valium, Librium, and Tranxene. Developed in the early 1960s, the benzodiazepines were considered safe substitutes for barbiturates, and the meprobamates (Miltown, Equanil). They act very quickly, particularly Valium. The calming effects are apparent within 30 minutes. Some of the benzodiazepines are long-acting (Valium, Librium, Tranxene, Klonopin, Centrax) and some are short-acting (Halcion, Ativan, Restoril). The main problem with these drugs is that they are habit forming, even at clinical dosages, and do have withdrawal symptoms so they are almost always avoided with the dually diagnosed patient for whom they can retrigger drug abuse. If the drug must be used, dosages are kept as low as possible and the patient is monitored for addiction or relapse.

Buspirone (BuSpar) is the only other drug labeled for generalized anxiety disorder. It is a serotonin modulator and will block the transmission of excess serotonin which is considered to be one of the causes of the symptoms of many forms of anxiety. It also mimics serotonin, so it can also substitute for low levels of serotonin, a feature used by some doctors to treat depression. It takes several weeks to work and is not nearly as initially dramatic as the benzodiazepines, so many patients are reluctant to use it. Its advantage, however, is that side effects are minimal and it is definitely not habit forming.

■ DRUGS FOR OBSESSIVE–COMPULSIVE DISORDER

For the obsessive–compulsive disorder almost every type of psychotropic medication has been used in the past, usually with relatively poor results. Anafranil (clomipramine) has recently been used with reasonable results. It is a serotonin reuptake inhibitor like Zoloft and Prozac.

■ DRUGS FOR PANIC DISORDER

Several drugs are used to control panic disorder (as opposed to panic attacks). Panic attacks occur in someone who has panic disorder, in those on a bad LSD trip, in someone having an extreme reaction to a stimulant, in a heart patient experiencing rapid heart beating (tachycardia), and in reactions to various medications. Panic disorder consists of multiple panic attacks accompanied by fear and anxiety about having more panic attacks. Situations where a panic attack might occur and they would be without help are also to be avoided. It is sometimes difficult to distinguish between a panic attack and a panic disorder.

Beta blockers calm the symptoms of a panic attack such as rapid heart rates, hypertension, and difficulty in breathing because they block excess muscular activity in the vascular system and lungs. Beta blockers also have a calming effect on the brain which is helpful in treating panic disorders. It takes about 1 hour for the medicine to work, so many people with a panic disorder or social phobia will take a dose 1 hour before entering a stressful situation.

The following list from Inaba and Cohen's outstanding book *Uppers, Downers, All-Arounders*[6] makes a handy reference to the categories discussed above:

MAJOR DEPRESSION
Tricyclic antidepressants: Imipramine (Tofranil, Janimine), desipramine (Norpramin, Pertofrane®), amitriptyline, (Elavil®, Endep), nortriptyline (Pamelor), Doxepin (Sinequan, Adapin®), trimipramine (Surmontil®), protriptyline (Vivactil®), maprotiline (Ludiomil®)
Monoamine oxidase (MAO) inhibitors: phenelzine (Nardil), tranylcypromine (Parnate), isocarboxazid (Marplan®), pargyline (Eutonyl®), belegiline (formerly Deprenyl now Eldepryl)
New antidepressants: fluoxetine (Prozac), trazodone (Desyrel), amoxapine (Asendin), alprazolam (benzodiazepine e.g., Xanax), bupropion (Welbutrin), sertraline (Zoloft), Ritanserin, paroxetine (Paxil®)

Stimulants used as antidepressants: amphetamines, Dexadrine, Biphetamine, Desoxyn, methylphenidate (Ritalin®), pemoline (Cylert)

BIPOLAR AFFECTIVE DISORDER (manic depression)
Lithium (Eskalith®, Lithobid®)
Others: Carbamazepine (Tegretol®), valproic acid (Depakene®), clonazepam (Klonopin®)

SCHIZOPHRENIA
Phenothiazines: trifluoperazine (Stelazine), fluphenazine (Proloxin, Permitil), perphenazine (Trilafon®), chlorpromazine (Thorazine), thioridazine (Mellaril), mesoridazine (Serentil®), triflupromazine (Vesprin), acetophenazine (Tindal), piperacetazine (Quide)
Others: halperidol (Haldol), thiothixene (Navane^V), loxapine (Loxitane), molindone (Moban, Lidone®), clozapine (Clozaril), pimozide (Orap), chlorprothixene (Taractan)

GENERALIZED ANXIETY DISORDER
Benzodiazepines
Short-acting (2–4 hour duration of action): alprazolam (Xanax), oxazepam (Serax), lorazepam (Ativan), triazolam (Halcion), temazepam (Restoril)
Long-acting (6–24 hour duration of action): diazepam (Valium), chlordiazepoxide (Librium), clorazepate (Tranxene), clonazepam (Klonopin), prazepam (Centrax), halazepam (Paxipam)
Non-benzodazepines: buspirone (BuSpar)

OBSESSIVE–COMPULSIVE DISORDER (OCD)
Clomipramine (Anafranil®), sertraline (Zoloft®), fluoxetine (Prozac®)

PANIC DISORDER
First-line drugs (medications which should be tried first to control panic): imipramine (Tofranil), desipramine (Norpramin or Pertofrane), alprazolam (Xanax)

Second-line drugs: phenelzine (Nardil), tranycypromine (Parnate), clonazepam (Klonopin)
Beta blockers: propranolol (Inderal), atenolol (Tenormin®)

SOCIAL PHOBIA
Beta blockers: propranolol (Inderal), atenolol (Tenormin)
MAO inhibitors: phenelzine (Nardil)

POSTTRAUMATIC STRESS SYNDROME
First-line drugs: benzodiazepines and sedatives in treatment of generalized anxiety disorder
Second-line drugs: antipsychotics as in the treatment of schizophrenia

SLEEPING DISORDER
Sleeping pills: flurazepam (Dalmane), triazolam (Halcion), temazepam (Restoril)

REFERENCES

1. Wartenberg AA: Management of common medical problems, in: Graham AW, Schultz TK, Wilford BB (eds.), *Principles of Addiction Medicine,* 2nd ed. Chevy Chase, MD: American Society of Addiction Medicine, 1998, p. 731.
2. Wartenberg AA: Medical syndromes associated with specific drugs, in: Graham AW, Schultz TK, Wilford BB (eds.), *Principles of Addiction Medicine,* 2nd ed. Chevy Chase, MD: American Society of Addiction Medicine, 1998, p. 809.
3. Cohen S, Gallant DM: Diagnosis of drug and alcohol abuse, in: Buchwald C, Katz D, Callahan JF (eds.), *Medical Monograph Series Volume 1, Number 6.* Brooklyn, NY: Career Teacher Center, State University of New York, 1981.
4. Seymour RB, Smith DE: *Physicians' Guide to Psychoactive Drugs.* Binghamton, NY: The Haworth Press, Inc., 1987.
5. Seymour RB, Smith DE: *The Psychedelic Resurgence: Treatment, Support, and Recovery Options.* Center City, MN: Hazelden, 1993.
6. Inaba D, Cohen WE: *Uppers, Downers, All Arounders,* 4th ed. Ashland, OR: CNS Productions, 2000.

7. Crome IB: Substance misuse and psychiatric comorbidity: towards improved service provisions. *Drugs: Education, Prevention and Policy, Source Id,* 1996; 6(2): 151–174.
8. Keller DS, Dermatis H: Current status of professional training in the addictions. *Substance Abuse: Journal of the Association for Medical Education and Research in Substance Abuse,* 1999; 20(3): 123–140.
9. Minkoff K, Regner J: Innovations in integrated dual diagnosis treatment in public managed care: the choat dial diagnosis case rate program. *Journal of Psychoactive Drugs,* 1999; 31(1): 3–12.

Chapter Nine

Treatment Issues Involving Family Dynamics

Statements to the effect that addiction only effects the addict are simply not true. The addict and drug abuser does not exist in a vacuum. Even the dedicated loner effects the lives of others, and most addicts live within some relationship to their families, friends, or coworkers.

Addiction is a Family Disease

Addiction affects families in many different ways, including shifting priorities and changing values, emergence of illness and disability, violence and exposure to other dangers, and enabling others to become victims of alcohol and other drugs. Addiction takes its toll on the human values that govern behavior, compromising the addicts investments of time, effort, and money.[1] Denial can open the door to dishonesty about one's drug-induced activities, and that dishonesty can be every bit as progressive as the addictive disease itself.

In the wake of the addiction, the family often practices its own forms of denial which can include the taking on of addiction dictated roles and developing a resigned acceptance, often including forms of manipulation by family members that throws the entire dynamic even more askew. There is a saying in the recovering community that in the addiction-based dysfunctional family there is an elephant in the living room. That elephant is the addiction, and nobody talks about it or even acknowledges that it is there, but all their actions and interactions function as a result of its presence.

Enabling and Enablers

Acting as though the most important priority is helping the active addict/alcoholic flourish on the short-term and prolong active addiction, is a good definition of what an enabler does. Enablers can include spouse, children, other family members, friends, and co-workers. Enabling behavior can take many forms and can be strongly influenced by both family structure, dictating roles within the family, and cultural factors, such as the strong relation in some cultures between alcohol abuse and domestic violence.

Wolin and colleagues[2,3] have pointed out that family rituals are influenced by and promote transmission of family cultural beliefs to future generations. Not only are there a wide variety of cultures of origin in the United States, but many families reflect mixed cultural backgrounds. Given such mixtures of cultural rules and beliefs, the protective elements that have been developed in the family members' cultural background can be deleted, producing a dissociation of rules about the use of alcohol and other drugs and associated behavior.

Family dynamics around addiction tend to be reactive, changing in response to the state of the addict at any given time. Much has been written about these dynamics, and in the 1980s a whole recovery literature grew up around the addict's dysfunctional family and the recovery of adult children of alcoholics and other addicts. Starting with Claudia Black's groundbreaking book *"It Will Never Happen to Me!,"*[4] which sold over 400,000 copies, young people throughout the United States self-identified as adult children of alcoholics and flocked to ACOA and ACA meetings.

The recovering community was early to recognize the plight of family in the dynamics of addiction. Early in the development of

Alcoholics Anonymous, the wives of its co-founders started the Family Group which evolved into Al-Anon and then begat Al Ateen as described in Chapter 7. Al-Anon and Al Ateen provide a forum for the family of alcoholics and addicts to work on the resultant family dysfunctions. The work and growth of Al-Anon was paralelled by the work of Joan Jackson, who studied and presented the stages of familial involvement in alcoholism as a developmental process.[5] By 1962, Ruth Fox was able to say, "Every member in such a family is affected emotionally, spiritually and in most cases economically, socially, and often physically."[6]

Around this time, the term "co-alcoholic" and then the more general "co-dependent" came into use to describe those individuals caught up in the interpersonal interaction with alcoholics and other addicts who responded with a reactive submissive response to the more domenent addict. Various researchers and clinicians expanded the focus beyond the primary alcoholic/addict to include the interactions, adjustments, and development of addict and family as a whole dynamic in and of itself, with parental alcoholism/addiction as a governing agent affecting the development of the family and its individuals.[7]

Stephanie Brown, one of the pioneers in family addiction treatment, has pointed out in lectures that the alcoholic family is not dysfunctional, it is functioning in its own way. It becomes dysfunctional when the alcoholic/addict enters treatment and begins to change out of the role that has been central and formative to the family. It is therefore a mistake to not take the family into full consideration in the course of treatment. Co-dependents need as much help and attention as the primary addict does. When the family structure as it is becomes threatened by the treatment and potential recovery of the primary addict, it may work to torpedo the process if steps are not taken to work with the family in transition.

Focusing on the alcoholic family in their chapter within the American Society of Addiction Medicine manual, *Principles of Addiction Medicine,* Brown and Lewis[7] present a dynamic for family recovery in which they contend that "The family follows a developmental progression from active drinking into transition, early recovery, and finally a stable, ongoing recovery, just like the alcoholic."[8]

Treating the Addictive Family

In her presentations at conferences in the 1980s, Sharon Wegscheider would develop a tableau on addictive family dynamics. First she would choose a volunteer from the audience to be the "addict/alcoholic," that person would stand on a chair so as to be "larger than life," then others from the audience would be selected to play spouse, children, friends, and co-workers. All of these would gather around the addict, leaning out of balance and drawn in by the dynamics of co-addiction. Then Sharon would remove the addict from the center for treatment, leaving a grotesque human construct. Then the addict would appear with a treatment chip shouting, "I'm free, I'm free!" But the tableau would still be there, would be what the treated individual was returning to. The message, of course, was that for treatment to succeed it had to involve the whole dynamic, at least the immediate family in its scope.[9]

Physicians and other health professionals have a unique potential for helping families deal with addictive disease. First of all, the family doctor or other health assessor can uncover the hidden problem, the invisible elephant. Clues can include ill-defined general complaints, unexplained trauma, psychic distress, and relationship problems. Intervention and referral, ranging from informal interaction with the family to a full, orchestrated professional intervention may follow in the efforts to introduce the addict into treatment. Physicians can continue to monitor the family situation, advising and providing guidance when appropriate throughout the process of treatment, transition, and recovery.[1]

Brown and Lewis[7] suggest a series of specific focus and treatment points for the drinking stage, the transitional stage, early recovery, and ongoing recovery. Although these are presented as specific to alcoholic familys, the same apply to the family dynamics involved in any substance addiction. During the drinking stage, movement toward treatment occurs when 1, 2, or more individuals from the above tableau begin to separate and detach from the unhealthy drinking environment. That is when the solidity of co-addiction begins to break up and dissolve.

The tasks of treatment in the drinking stage include:

- To challenge the behaviors and thinking that maintain the pathology of the environment, the system, and the individuals.
- To help family members shift focus from the system to themselves.
- To encourage and provide support for detachment and separation.

In the transition stage, when the alcoholic/addict is in the process of transiting from active addiction to active recovery, the therapist can help the family to focus on:

- breaking denial;
- realizing that family life is out of control;
- beginning a challenge of core beliefs;
- hitting bottom and surrender;
- accepting the reality of alcoholism and loss of control;
- allowing the alcoholic system to collapse;
- shifting the focus from the system to the individuals who begin detachment and individual recovery;
- enlisting outside supports, such as A.A., Al-Anon, Alateen, and professional treatment; and
- learning new abstinent behaviors and thinking.

The tasks of treatment in this transional state include working with the family to:

- To challenge denial and offer support for movement into recovery for all individuals.
- To support a shift in focus off the family system and on to the individuals.

- To add supports such as AA, Al-Anon, etc., outside the family.
- To include parenting responsibilities and help parents structure their recoveries to fulfill them.

In the early recovery stage, when abstinence, new thinking, attitudes, and behavior are taking place, the therapist needs to help the family focus on:

- Continuing to learn abstinent behaviors and thinking.
- Stabilizing individual identities: I am an alcoholic, I am a co-alcoholic, and I have lost control.
- Continuing close contact with Twelve Step programs and working the steps.
- Maintaining a focus on individual recovery, seeking supports outside the family.
- Continuing detachment and a limited family focus.
- Maintaining parenting responsibilities.

Treatment tasks during this same early recovery stage include:

- Continuing to attend to behavior and cognitive change.
- Solidifying and building identities as alcoholic and co-alcoholic.
- Supporting individual focus; using couples therapy to help couples tolerate separation.
- Supporting Twelve Step programs and helping with resistance.
- Maintaining recovery assessment and watcing for signs of relapse.
- Supporting parenting responsibilities.
- Facilitating insight-oriented psychotherapy or trauma resolution as necessary.

Ongoing recovery solidifies abstinence and the development of a drug-free life, the development of new interests and expanding horizons. A spiritual focus develops that involves connectedness and relinquishing of control, a letting go of manipulative control behaviors by both the addict and the co-addicts. Families can lay the foundation for a new, healthy relationship that involves finding a balance between individual, couple and family growth. At this point the therapist's job is to help the family:

- Continue abstinent behavior.
- Continue to build alcoholic and co-alcoholic identities.
- Maintain individual programs of recovery; to continue to work the Twelve Steps and internalize the Twelve Step principles.
- Work through the consequences of alcoholism and co-alcoholism to the self and family.
- Deepen spirituality.
- Add a focus on couple and family issues.
- Balance and integrate combined individual and family recoveries.[10]

Family Treatment

Due to the efforts of such individuals as Sharon Wegscheider,[9] Stephanie Brown and Virginia Lewis, most residential addiction programs now have family components. Family members at these treatment centers may attend similar lectures on recovery and many treatment protocols now include an intensive Family Week when spouses and even other family members live at the facility for a time, although they may be kept separate from the family member in addiction treatment for most of that time while they work on their own co-dependence and recovery issues.[11]

Since the 1980s, a variety of family systems therapy approaches have been developed that integrate family systems therapy and addiction treatment, often including the concurrent use of AA and Al-Anon. Mark Galanter has developed a network therapy that combines direct work with the addict and a few signif-icant members of the family or social system with participation in Twelve Step Programs and the prescription of disulfiram or naltrexone.[12] Two well-developed behavioral approaches to marital alcoholism treatment are the Program for Alcoholic Couples Treatment (PACT)[13] and Counseling for Alcoholics' Marriages (CALM)[14]. PACT involves 15 couples sessions with homework and self-monitored exercises in between. Alcoholic and spouse behavior is modified through stimulus control procedures, contingency rearrangement, cognitive restructuring, a functional analysis of the drinking, techniques to stop triggering and reinforcing drinking, and the development of alternatives, with communications training emphasizing problem solving and negotiating skills. CALM involves 6–8 prep sessions, then 10 multiple couples' group meetings that feature discussion on preventing and dealing with relapse, communications and negotiations skills training and positive family activities.

In general, an integrated approach that conbines the warmth and appeal of disease model approaches, the scope of family systems approaches and the scientific rigor of behavioral approaches may ultimately be the key to successful family addiction treatment.[11]

REFERENCES

1. Liepman MR: The family in addiction, in: Graham AW, Schultz TK, Wilford BB (eds.), *Principles of Addiction Medicine,* 2nd ed. Chevy Chase, MD: American Society of Addiction Medicine, 1998; p. 1093.
2. Wolin SJ, Bennett LA, Noonan DL: Family rituals and the recurrence of alcoholism over generations. *American Journal of Psychiatry,* 1979; 136(4B): 589–593.
3. Wolen SJ, Bennett LA, Noonan DL, Teitelbaum MA: Disrupted family rituals: a factor in the intergenerational transmission of alcoholism. *Journal of Studies on Alcohol,* 1980; 41: 199–214.
4. Black C: *"It Will Never Happen to Me!"* New York, NY: Ballantine Books, 1987.
5. Jackson J: The adjustment of the family to the crisis of alcoholism. *Quarterly Journal of Studies on Alcohol,* 1954; 15: 562–586.
6. Fox R: Children in the alcoholic family, in: Bier WC (ed.), *Problems in Addiction: Alcoholism and Narcotics.* New York, NY: Fordham University Press, 1962.

7. Brown S, Lewis V: A developmental model of the alcoholic family, in: Graham AW, Schultz TK, Wilford BB (eds.), *Principles of Addiction Medicine,* 2nd ed. Chevy Chase, MD: American Society of Addiction Medicine, 1998, p. 1099.
8. Brown S: *Treating the Alcoholic: A Developmental Model of Recovery.* New York, NY: John Wiley & Sons, 1985.
9. Wegscheider S: *Another Chance: Hope and Health for the Alcoholic Family.* Palo Alto, CA: Science & Behavior Books, 1981.
10. Brown S, Lewis V: *Maintaining Abstinence Program: A Curriculum for Families in Recovery.* Palo Alto, CA: Mental Research Institute, Family Recovery Project, 1993.
11. Berenson D, Schrier EW: Current family treatment approaches, in: Graham AW, Schultz TK, Wilford BB (eds.), *Principles of Addiction Medicine,* 2nd ed. Chevy Chase, MD: American Society of Addiction Medicine, 1998, p. 1115.
12. Galanter M: Network therapy, in: Graham AW, Schultz TK, Wilford BB (eds.), *Principles of Addiction Medicine,* 2nd ed. Chevy Chase, MD: American Society of Addiction Medicine, 1998, p. 653.
13. Noel NS, McCrady BS: Alcohol-focused spouse involvement with behavioral marital therapy, in: TJ O'Farrell (ed.), *Treating Alcoholic Problems: Marital and Family Interventions.* New York, NY: Guilford Press, 1993.
14. O'Farrell TJ: A behavioral marital therapy couples group program for alcoholics and their spouses, in: TJ O'Farrell (ed.), *Treating Alcoholic Problems: Marital and Family Interventions.* New York, NY: Guilford Press, 1993.

10

Women in Treatment: Addiction, Abuse, and Pregnancy and Treating Elderly Patients

Up until the last decade, serious study of addiction and substance abuse was primarily focused on the male population, while data on women was either discarded or generalized to both sexes. Treatment approaches were also male oriented. For many years, it was assumed that alcohol and other drugs would have the same effects on women as they had on men. The fact is that addicted women differ from men in a number of important ways and have quite different needs in treatment.

Differences between male and female addict populations are both physiological and sociocultural. For example, when given equal doses of alcohol, women reach higher peak blood alcohol concentrations as a result of higher levels of alcohol dehydrogenase (ADH) in men's gastric mucosa. This leads to a more active first-pass metabolism within the stomach wall and less absorption.[1] Women's higher proportion of body fat also produces differences in drug reaction.

Long-term heavy drinking by women has been associated with a variety of reproductive dysfunctions, such as inhibition of ovulation, decrease in gonadal mass, irregular menses, luteal phase dysfunction and early menopause.[2]

According to Blume,[3] although both men and women are subject to many serious medical complications from heavy drinking and other drug use, such problems as fatty liver, hypertension, anemia, malnutrition, gastrointestinal (GI) hemorrhage, peripheral myopathy and peptic ulcer may develop more rapidly in women. Breast cancer may be related to alcohol abuse. The incidence of AIDS in women has been steadily increasing. According to a Center on Addiction and Substance Abuse study,[4] 70% of AIDS cases in women are related to substance abuse, half from personal injection drug use and another quarter sexually transmitted from injection drug users.

In general, women use less alcohol and illegal drugs than men but use more prescription psychoactives. This may be iatrogenic to the extent that women have been a prime population for the overprescribing of sedatives.

Identification and Assessment of Women with Substance Abuse

Denial is often stronger for women than it is for men. Women tend to be hidden drinkers and users, stigmatized by their activity and kept out of treatment by individual and family denial. If pregnant, they may avoid treatment because of the stringent penalties that may include loss of children. Many women addicts are victims of childhood and sexual abuse and may be battered as adults.

Use for women often begins later than that of men, but addiction will develop more rapidly and treatment entry is at about the same time. Women addicts are more likely to be married or living with an alcoholic or addicted sexual partner or to be divorced or separated. While the quantity of alcohol or other drug intake may be lower than it usually is for men, the disease is every bit as serious. Women are more likely than men to suffer from dual diagnosis, exhibiting psychiatric symptoms as well as addictive disease. Unlike men who usually seek treatment as a result of problems at work or with the law, women seek treatment primarily through mental and physical health problems and problems with family members.

Drugs and Procreation

Drugs and procreation have become an increasingly important issue, particularly with the identification of Fetal Alcohol Syndrome and notoriety of "crack babies." It is clear that many psychoactive drugs have marked teratogenic effect, making use of drugs during pregnancy a critical issue, and in some parts of the United States grounds for at times draconian measures against women who have used alcohol and other drugs during pregnancy.

The reaction to lurid tales of crack babies and the increasing recognition of FAS and other neonatal drug syndromes has at times included the advocating that women who are using be jailed through term and/or face major legal approbation. Such overreaction runs counter to public health reality in that its primary result is to keep women who need it from seeking pre-natal care and thereby putting their unborn child at even greater risk. Drug use by an expectant mother is a highly complex medical issue. Withdrawal during pregnancy may be entirely the wrong answer, placing the fetus at great risk.[5]

Concern in such cases is well founded. The use of drugs, including alcohol, during pregnancy has been clearly related to increased morbidity and mortality for the mother, the fetus, and the subsequent infant.[6] That risk can be decreased however with identification of the problem and adequate, knowledgable prenatal and natal care, which at best should be provided by a physician who is both knowledgeable about high risk obstetrics and addiction medicine, or through a team that provides such combined knowledge.

The question of whether and/or how to detoxify an expectant mother during pregnancy must take into account both the effects of withdrawal on the mother but on the fetus and neonate. Detailed guidelines for prenatal detoxification and treatment are available from the federal Center for Substance Abuse Treatment (CSAT),[7] which advises that initial stabilization should be accomplished within 10 days of first contact or earlier if medically needed. Stabilization should always precede any attempt at detoxification. It should always be kept in mind that withdrawal, particularly from alcohol and other sedative type drugs can be life-threatening in and of itself if badly handled or if complications take place.

A Brief History of Women's Treatment Efforts

Women-centered treatment for drug problems had a varied history, most recently starting up as an aspect of the women's health movement in the 1960s. In the fall of 1970, a war on drugs treatment grant from the federal government allowed the Haight Ashbury Free Clinics in San Francisco to initiate a drug abuse detoxification, rehabilitation and aftercare project with its own building and a paid staff. Two young women, Kish Stefko and Jeannie Kubiki, who had been providing drug counseling at the old site in the Clinics' medical program, asked for a room in the new building where they could provide a range of services specifically for women drug clients. These services included venereal disease screening, rape counseling, and abortion counseling and referral along with standard drug counseling. The basic philosophy these counselors espoused was that of women helping women in health matters that were deeply personal.[8]

The new women's consciousness found paternalism and other judgmental facets of male-dominated medicine just as objectionable as the counter culture in general had found traditional medicine a few years earlier. The publication of *Our Bodies, Our Selves*,[9] a women's health guide, had promoted the consciousness that medical self-knowledge was a form of personal empowerment. Women were now looking to programs empathetic with their needs and feelings, not what male clinicians thought women should need and feel. The need was particularly acute in the treatment of addiction, where women were coming into treatment from situations that made them highly vulnerable and in dire need of special treatment.

■ BARRIERS TO TREATMENT FOR WOMEN

Women face a number of barriers to treatment for their drug addiction problems. The absence of adequate child care makes residential treatment virtually impossible for any mother who has no resources for taking care of their children and who risk losing them if they enter into treatment that takes them away from the home. This problem is particularly acute in that many female addicts are divorced or separated mothers. As mentioned earlier in this chapter, women also face the threat of losing their children on legal grounds in many states and communities. Legal definitions that equate drug addiction with child abuse or neglect may put an addicted mother at risk of custody loss if she asks for assistance with child care or even attempts to enter residential drug treatment.[10]

Above and beyond the risk of custody loss, women in the 1990s and beyond also faced the threat of civil or criminal prosecution.

Barriers to treatment for women can also be financial. Because they tend to be unemployed or work in low paying jobs that do not provide benefits, single mothers often lack insurance coverage for treatment.

In the 1980s, the federal Center for Substance Abuse Prevention launched a number of women-specific treatment projects throughout the United States and many of these included facilities that could accommodate a woman and her children. The CSAP grants were unfortunately short-term and when the funding ran out many of these efforts had to be curtailed for lack of fiscal support.

Focusing on Problems of the Elderly

As more is being learned about women in addiction, another population is coming into focus and that is the elderly. At a time when the "baby boom" is moving into its own '60s, there is more interest and concern for the issues that are particular to an aging population that has tended to be ignored heretofore. The following represents some notes and guidelines on substance abuse and addiction issues that are specific to an aging population.

■ PATTERNS OF ABUSE

Although this is changing as veterans of the Age of Rock and Roll collect their AARP membership cards, in general the older drug addict/abuser is not part of a cohesive illicit drug culture. By and large, drug abuse in older adults has had iatrogenic origins. Similar to the middle-class polydrug abuser first identified and studied by David Smith and Don Wesson in the 1970s, drugs of abuse for the older adult tend toward prescription pharmaceuticals, usually prescribed by a variety of physicians, and alcohol.[11]

By contrast, the using careers of street-drug users within drug using subcultures usually end—either in death or abstinence—before the aging process is well under way. One rarely sees what used to be the real meaning of "an old geezer." Heroin users who survive tend to reach a point where they can no longer cope with the often hectic process of procuring and using their drug and either enter treatment or manage to stop.

On the other hand, an increasingly evident phenomenon is the life-long maintenance alcoholic, usually someone well situated in the business world, who blossoms into full abuse after retirement. These individuals may have masked their use during their working career through heavy workloads. They have helpers to bolster their denial system and manage until they find themselves no longer surrounded by sycophantic employees and co-workers and can no longer hold their disease in check with a precipitous work-pace. Instead, with little but time on their hands and surrounded by a loving family that has only seen them for short periods of time in the past, their disease blossoms.

The increased attention on the elderly has shown, however, that there are physiological factors involved in the differences between the aging and younger abusers. James W. Smith[12] points out that age-related factors in alcohol metabolism include a decrease in the gastric alcohol dehydrogenase enzyme (ADH), the enzyme responsible for initiating the metabolism of alcohol in the gastric mucosa.

Long-Term Effects of Tobacco and Alcohol

Tobacco produces the most deadly long-term effects, including lung, mouth esophagus and other cancers, potentially fatal cardio-vascular, circulatory and respiratory disease. Presently, tobacco is responsible for over 400,000 deaths a year in the United States alone. One doesn't even have to be particularly old to die from the effects of tobacco.

The combination of alcohol and tobacco can produce a double-barrel negative effect on the immune system, while alcohol has its own degenerative effects over time. In his American Society of Addiction Medicine chapter, Smith also discusses the many long-term effects of alcohol that may become evident in the older adult. Essentially, alcohol is a particularly virulent toxin when it is used to excess over long periods of time, and as such can have a deleterious effect on many parts of the body. These include:

- The brain: brain atrophy and dementia.
- Pharynx: cancer, increasing 10-fold in drinkers who also smoke.
- Esophagus: esophagitis and esophageal varices.
- Heart: alcoholic cardiomyopathy, reversible only in early stages.
- Lungs: lowered resistance can lead to tuberculosis, pneumonia and emphysema.
- Liver: cirrhosis, acute and irreversible enlargement among other problems.
- Spleen: Hypersplenism.
- Stomach: gastritis and ulcers.
- Pancreas: acute and chronic pancreatitis.
- Testes: atrophy.

- Long nerves: Peripheral neuropathy, generally reversible and characterized by loss of sensation, weakness and pain.
- Muscles: alcoholic myopathy.
- Blood and bone marrow: coagulation defects and anemia.

■ PSYCHIATRIC EFFECTS

Besides the physical effects of alcohol and other drugs on the older adult, there are also greater vulnerabilities to psychiatric compli-cations. For example, withdrawal can be more harrowing with alcoholic delirium tremens and corresponding effects from other drug withdrawal being more pronounced in the older adult. Depression and suicide are other key results of long-term use and the aging process.

Need To Know When Medicating the Older Adult

In general, the clinician needs to be aware that for a variety of phy-siological reasons older individuals who are being medicated with psychoactive medications should be given much lower doses than younger patients. For example, the effective dose of a benzo-diazepine for a 70-year-old may be less than half that called for in a 40-year-old patient.

Older patients tend to have tremendous trust in their health providers and also tend to not ask questions when they really need to. The clinician is left with the task of anticipating what an older patient needs to know and how to provide information to a segment of the population that sees physicians as all wise and all powerful. For example, older patients often are given prescrip-tions by their primary-care provider as well as a variety of specia-lists over time. Often, if they are not told to stop using a given medication, they don't. Also they may be taking medications that have dangerous cross-tolerance or should not be taken with one another. Also, they may be taking long-term medications at doses that are no longer appropriate. The clinician who is the primary-care giver should review the medications that older patients are taking on a regular basis and discuss what effects the patient is experiencing.

REFERENCES

1. Frezza M, di Padova C, Pozzato G, Terpin M, Baraona E, Lieber CS: High blood alcohol levels in women: the role of decreased gastric alcohol dehydrogenase activity and first-pass metabolism. *The New England Journal of Medicine,* 1990; 322(2): 95–99.
2. Mello NK: Drug use and premenstrual dysphoria, in: BA Ray, MC Braude (eds.), *Women and Drugs: A New Era for Research (NIDA Monograph 65)* Rockville, MD: National Institute on Drug Abuse, 1986.
3. Blume SB: Understanding addictive disorders in women, in: Graham AW, Schultz TK, Wilford BB (eds.), *Principles of Addiction Medicine,* 2nd ed. Chevy Chase, MD: American Society of Addiction Medicine, 1998, p. 1173.
4. Center on Addiction and Substance Abuse: *Substance Abuse and American Women.* New York, NY: CASA, 1996.
5. Smith DE, Lusher T, Seymour RB: Benzodiazepines and other sedative-hypnotic withdrawal, in: M Jessup (ed.), *Drug Dependency in Pregnancy: Managing Withdrawal.* North Highlands, CA: State of California Department of General Services, 1992.
6. Miller LJ: Treatment of the addicted woman in pregnancy, in: Graham AW, Schultz TK, Wilford BB (eds.), *Principles of Addiction Medicine,* 2nd ed. Chevy Chase, MD: American Society of Addiction Medicine, 1998, p. 1199.
7. Center for Substance Abuse Treatment: *Treatment Improvement Protocol for Pregnant, Substance-Using Women.* Rockville, MD: CSAT, 1993.
8. Seymour RB, Smith DE: *The Haight Ashbury Free Clinics: Still Free After All These Years.* San Francisco: Partisan Press, 1986.
9. Boston Women's Health Collective: *Our Bodies, Our Selves.* New York, NY: Simon & Schuster, 1969.
10. Blume SB: Women and alcohol: issues in social policy, in: RW Wilsnack, SC Wilsnack (eds.), *Gender and Alcohol.* Piscataway, NJ: Rutgers Center of Alcohol Studies, 1997.

11. Smith DE, Wesson DR, Seymour RB: The abuse of barbiturates and other sedative hypnotics, in: DuPont RI, Goldstein A, O'Donnel (eds.), *Handbook of Drug Abuse*. Washington DC: National Institute on Drug Abuse and White House Office on Drug Abuse Policy, 1979.

12. Smith JW: Special problems of the elderly, in: Graham AW, Schultz TK, Wilford BB (eds.), *Principles of Addiction Medicine,* 2nd ed. Chevy Chase, MD: American Society of Addiction Medicine, 1998, p. 833.

Chapter Eleven

Treating Children and Adolescents

What is it like to be a teenager involved in alcohol and other drugs at the start of the new millennium? Speaking at an American Society of Addiction Medicine (ASAM) Medical Conference on Adolescent Addictions, David E. Smith, M.D., presented a startling scenario in the spectrum of adolescent drug abuse and addiction. Dr. Smith's presentation followed an actors-on-videotape enhanced exposition by a suburban, white pediatrician of the problems involved in working with a sulky white teenager, his distraught mother, and attempts at engaging the so so busy yuppie businessman father in the problem. Taking his place at the podium, Dr. Smith lauded that speaker for presenting one aspect of adolescent drug problems and stated his own case:

> At the Haight Ashbury Clinics, we do a lot of work with inner-city African-Americans in San Francisco and the East Bay. In these settings, we see a far different family picture. The mother is not trying to dominate the pediatrician. There is no pediatrician and the mother is too far gone on crack cocaine herself to care. The father is most likely doing hard time in the penitentiary. The adolescent client and his or her peers are out in the streets, selling crack and shooting at each other with automatic weapons. The only relatively stable element is often the grandmother, who is doing her best to try and keep some semblance of a family together and dreading the arrival of the mother's next crack cocaine-affected baby.

While Dr. Smith's presentation obviously represents a worst-case scenario, variations on the theme he has described are by no means limited to minority populations and the desperately poor. Within the spectrum of adolescent treatment, it soon becomes obvious that the worst problems arise from unwholesome societal and family situations, which may be at their most obvious among the poor, but from which the rich and the middle-class are far from immune.

There has been a decrease in the number of adolescents entering treatment. Positive reasons for that decrease include the effectiveness of school and community prevention programs, recognition and intervention that brings younger abusers into treatment earlier in their abuse, and an increasingly negative attitude toward drug use, including alcohol and tobacco, among the educated and the affluent. Less positive reasons may include a decrease in availability of treatment facilities for adolescents whose families cannot afford expensive care and government policies that have emphasized incarceration rather than treatment for young drug users. More young people are showing up in the criminal justice system. Roughly 80% of individuals currently serving time in federal, state and local prison facilities are on charges that involve substance abuse, while less than 5% are in treatment.[1]

There may be fewer young people entering alcohol and drug dependency treatment, but according to the professionals who treat them, those that do seem to be "getting sicker." As the overall number of young people entering treatment continues to decrease, the shared experience of the counselors and therapists who work with them is that their presenting problems are becoming more intractable. While the relative number of young people entering treatment is declining, the age of first use is getting lower as well, making alcohol and other drug problems in youth more severe and more difficult to treat. Additionally, young people enter treatment today with multiple problems, including severe learning disorders, borderline personality disorders and other problems related to dual diagnosis, and issues arising out of child abuse and molestation. They also present much more difficult family histories of alcoholism and other addictions that create greater dysfunction within the family.

There is an enormous rate of relapse among teenagers. The public does not see relapse as part of the recovery process. Relapse is seen as failure, failure is remembered more readily than success. Whether treatment is paid for privately, reimbursed by health insurance, or funded by local, state or federal government, it is costly and getting more so each year. In an effort to curtail expenses, insurance companies and other third-party payers are less willing to foot the bill. In the private sector, an increasing number of adolescent programs are closing and many existing beds remain unfilled. At the same time, in the public sector waiting lists are long and services often nonexistent, while social justice issues such as poverty, illiteracy, and racism related to alcohol and other drug problems continue unabated. An example of social injustice can be seen in the response to a perceived proliferation of drug-impaired babies that has occurred in some inner-city areas where public money has been used to facilitate taking these babies away from their mothers rather than providing funding for treatment.

All of these factors have made it increasingly difficult for physicians and therapists to work with adolescents. These problems tax our patience and test the very limits of our experience, and indeed, our confidence. Professionals who work with adolescents have had to deal with increasing threats of violence, threats of suicide, a growing number of cases involving self-inflicted wounds and mutilation, the phenomena of cult and gang membership, and other issues that were much less common in the past.

Training programs for professionals who have chosen to work with adolescents are often inadequate to the task of dealing with these issues. There are some in-service programs dealing specifically with such issues as the threat of violence at the treatment site, but these programs often lack effective attitudinal training.

Most of the adolescent treatment programs across the country with which the authors are familiar employ the 12 Steps pioneered by Alcoholics Anonymous as a central theme and as the foundation for recovery. Many professionals are engaged as active members in 12-Step programs themselves, and endeavor to apply these principles to their work on a daily basis. In the midst of pressure and stress, however, it is often easy to forget that *it is not so much what we teach young people, but the example that we set that is most effective.* Who we are is as important as what we teach. The environment that we create, and the nature of the consciousness that we hold has as great an effect as our treatment philosophies. If we can maintain an awareness that the patient is teaching us as we teach them, a meeting can take place beyond the roles that we assume and project.

As youngsters come to treatment who do in fact have multiple problems and greater difficulties, the tendency is to treat them by rote. The use of a standard set of rules and procedures, the power of our authority or the lever of the authority of courts becomes a more tempting and a more prevalent approach. It is much more difficult to engage not only in a professional clinical practice, but a practice of personal, spiritual recovery; whether it is our own recovery from an addiction to substances or the recognition of our co-dependency created out of the very nature of our work. Added to this dilemma is the fact that many counselors and therapists who choose to work with adolescents have had the same problems when they were young. We bring forward the aspects of ourselves that are as yet unhealed, regardless of how long we have "been in the program," regardless of how much training we have had or how much we may know or think we know. The process of our recovery is lifelong.

If we pay attention to our work, we will notice that we often swing between two poles. On the one hand, we enjoy the feeling of being "on top of it," knowing just what we are doing. We possess a sense of mastery and self-confidence. Then there are times when we become particularly stuck and feel as if we know nothing at all and have no right to be practicing therapists. We become all but overwhelmed with feelings of incompetence, believing we are impostors. In her paper, *The Wounded Healer: Power and Vulnerability in the Psychotherapy Relationship,* Amy Weston[2] says that she "began to recognize a theme about the extreme discomfort and the feelings of uselessness and help-lessness that are evoked in a therapist. A discomfort to a point that defensive behaviors emerge in order to feel less wounded." Her supervisees were reporting attacks on their capacity to be helpful or nurturing which she also recognized in herself. Alice Miller, in her book *Prisoners of Childhood*,[3] describes the narcis-sistic injuries that bring people into the helping professions. She says that many people seek the helping professions in an attempt to heal the wounds or injuries that were created in childhood. Amy Weston[2] also states that, "the need to be the helper and to institutionalize the role by entering a helping profession can be seen as an important personal motivation and as a collective wound of the profession." She says that " . . . it began to seem as if the experience of one's powerlessness as a therapist came with the territory. That the therapist's experience of uncertainty, helplessness, and occasional uselessness was an integral part of the process of healing."

If these statements are true, or if we are willing to entertain them as being possibly true for the purpose of this discussion, the direction in which they point is an important consideration for working with adolescents. It is hard to imagine any other type of client that poses the kinds of difficulties the adolescent pre-sents. A majority of the young people who enter treatment for chemical dependency have one or both parents who are alcoholic or drug dependent (estimates range from 60–65%). Although many parents who intervene upon their child's addiction are in recovery themselves, most are still in denial about their own addiction. Often related to or as a result of parental addiction, there is a history of family violence including psychological and physical abuse, molestation, and incest. Unlike the adult who can choose to leave, the adolescent is trapped in this dysfunc-tional, sometimes brutal family system that lacks true intimacy. And often growing out of all of this is the impact of poor educa-tional and vocational skills. The teenager must struggle to deal with all the issues of being chemically dependent and the co-dependent child of an alcoholic/addict concurrently. Not only is the teenager suffering from the effects of alcoholism and other drug addiction but, as Timmen Cermak has pointed out,[4] they suffer from the effects of post-traumatic stress disorder (PTSD). The young addict/alcoholic has grown up in the "war zone," they are "shell shocked."

There are two common errors in working with adolescent clients. The first of these is trying to become the patient's friend. This results in the undermining of authority. The therapist becomes an enabler, thereby exacerbating the problem by eroding therapeutic effectiveness. The second is becoming rigid and not allowing a therapeutic relationship to develop. This is the therapist as authoritarian and disciplinarian, locking the client out and becoming abusive in the relationship. The question, then, is how can one be empathetic without falling prey to these two extremes?

An approach to an answer is possible if the therapist is willing to develop an understanding of what spiritual, biochemical, psychological, social, and cultural forces are at work in distressed adolescents who are experiencing alcohol and other drug problems. Where is the line, for example, between willful obstruction and helpless denial? Is the adolescent an addict who is prey to all the disease symptomatology that is at work in the adult addict? Or is the young substance abuser the subject of a totally different etiology?[5]

Current Trends in Adolescent Drug Abuse

It has been observed that adolescents are the only age group in the United States whose morbidity and mortality rates have worsened over the past 30 years. For example, one-fourth of adolescents contract a sexually transmitted disease before they graduate from high school. Further, a smaller percentage of teens are graduating from high school today than were in 1985. At present, a full 5% of 16-to-19-year-olds are idle: they are not in school, not in the labor force, not in the military, and not homemakers. The fact that such large numbers of teens have no productive role in society has obvious implications for delinquency, neighborhood stability, and youth alienation.[6]

Current Drug Trends Among Adolescents

Today's youth has an expanded pharmacopoeia of relatively accessible licit and illicit drugs to choose from, and little to prevent experimentation and the slide into abuse. Even though the dangers of smoking tobacco are more clearly known and the incidence of early-onset alcoholism is rising, parents are often relieved to find that their children are using alcohol and tobacco rather than illicit drugs, and may actually encourage their use. Look-alike drugs, made from such non-scheduled substances as caffeine, ephedrine, and phenylpropanolamine (PPA) are manufactured to look like powerful prescription stimulants. These form a border-zone between the licit and illicit drugs and can produce dangerous side effects when taken in enough quantity to provide a psychoactive rush.

Several of the illicit drugs favored by adolescents have undergone transformations that make them more potent, while others have become increasingly available to the youth market:

- *Crack cocaine* is a combination of cocaine hydrochloride and baking soda that can be produced in specific doses. Easy to transport and sell in small quantities, crack is smoked, delivering a highly potent dose directly to the brain through the lungs. Although the price of a single unit may be low, compulsive use rapidly makes this an expensive habit that adolescents can only maintain by selling crack themselves.

- *Ice* is a smokable form of methamphetamine, another highly potent stimulant with a massive entry comparable to that of crack but with effects lasting hours instead of minutes.

- *Hybrid forms of marijuana*, such as "sinsemilla," contain many times the active ingredient, delta-9-tetrahydrocannabinol (THC), than is found in even the most potent forms of naturally occurring cannabis.

- *Psilocybin*, the "magic" mushrooms that were a rare hallucinogen in the 1970s, are now cultivated throughout the country and readily available.
- *LSD,* the "psychedelic" drug of the 1960s is now being used in higher dosages by adolescents after a lower-dose hiatus.
- *MDMA, GHB, Rohypnol* and other party drugs are used at "raves" and other teen gatherings. Both GHB and rohypnol or "roofies" have gained a reputation as "date rape" drugs, used to render women semi-conscious by predatory males.
- *Phencyclidine (PCP)*, a mind/body disassociative drug that acts like a stimulant, sedative-hypnotic or hallucinogen depending on dosage, can have extremely debilitating long-term effects, is still the drug of choice in many adolescent groups, while other drugs such as heroine, designer opioids, and a variety of prescription stimulants and sedative-hypnotic drugs usually associated with adult use often find their way into the hands and brains of adolescents.

The Adolescent Drug User

Young people who are in treatment are often using alcohol and other drugs to get high on a daily basis. Also, they started younger than their 20th century predecessors. In the year 2000, the current age of onset in California ranges from 11.7 years all the way down to 8.8 years. When a young person begins to use that early and has a biochemical pre-disposition to compulsion, the dilemma is compounded.

The basics of the addictive disease model are the same for pre-adolescents, adolescents and adults. By its tenets, addiction is a disease in and of itself, creating its own psychopathology and characterized by compulsion, loss of control, and continued use in spite of adverse consequences. Addictive disease is chronic, progressive, and potentially fatal if not treated. At present, there is no known cure. It can be brought into remission, however, through abstinence from all psychoactive drugs and supported recovery.[7]

Beyond these basics, however, it is counterproductive to overlay adult models on adolescent drug users. Physiologically, adolescents are at high risk for early onset addiction with the risk increasing the younger use is initiated. Psychologically, adolescents may consider themselves to be indestructible and tend to be unconcerned about long-term dangers of drugs. Educational descriptions of drug consequences often backfire, creating a seduction and enticing youth into experimentation rather than warning them away from use.

Prevention

In the overall schematic of adolescent substance abuse, prevention is often cited as the all-encompassing concept. One speaks of "primary, secondary and tertiary prevention." What this means is: primary prevention is aimed at those who are at risk but have not used drugs; secondary prevention is aimed at those who have experimented with drugs but not abused them; and tertiary prevention is aimed at those who are abusing drugs but are not chemically dependent. Yet another aspect of prevention is that of relapse prevention.

Prevention is the task of the community as a whole, but physicians can play a key role in prevention education and secondary and tertiary intervention. This role involves education of both adolescent patients and their parents regarding the nature of drug abuse and how it happens within a family dynamic. In providing such counseling it helps to have a concept of not only current prevention modalities but of future possibilities as well.

The Relation of Primary Prevention to Treatment......................

Many individuals, including many health professionals, do not have a clear idea of prevention, particularly primary prevention, and its relationship to treatment. In their books, *Drugfree: A Unique, Positive Approach to Staying Off Alcohol and Other Drugs,*[7] and *The New Drugs: Look-Alikes, Drugs of Deception and Designer Drugs,* Seymour et al.[8] present an image defining primary prevention and go on to discuss some innovative approaches to prevention.

Imagine that there is a bridge over a river. During a storm, the center span of the bridge has collapsed. Cars continue to drive onto the bridge and when they reach the middle they fall through into the river. Now a rescue effort has been mounted. Volunteers dive into the river downstream, haul the survivors out of their cars and do their best to resuscitate these victims. There is a lot of traffic, so a tremendous effort is needed to reach all the cars that float by. That is treatment.

One of the rescuers suggests that someone climb up to the road on both sides of the river and put up signs warning drivers that the bridge is out. Perhaps some effort should also be put into working out a detour around the bridge. That is primary prevention.

Primary prevention consists of any means that leads an adolescent or pre-adolescent to voluntarily avoid abuse of drugs or any other dangerous activity. Recognized prevention strategies include education, inducement, conditioning and preventional alternatives, to name a few. Sometimes prevention involves one individual and sometimes a group, such as a class in school or a whole society. Some prevention measures have involved the development of employment opportunities for poverty-level groups whose precarious socioeconomic position makes them particularly vulnerable to the "panacea" of drug abuse. Others involve creating teen centers or special projects that increase self-worth and provide drug-free activities.

Although virtually everyone thinks that primary drug- and alcohol-abuse prevention is necessary and a good idea, it is often a stepchild to treatment, an activity that is hard to implement and fund. This is not surprising in a society where physical results tend to mean so much. While treatment statistics, cure rates and arrest records are manipulated to support the "fact" that something is being accomplished, it is awfully hard to show how many young people are *not* using drugs as a result of primary prevention efforts. And yet there is general agreement that keeping young people from abusing alcohol and other drugs in the first place is our highest substance-abuse priority.

There are differing opinions on what constitutes effective substance-abuse prevention. The approaches based on these opinions have developed through recent decades, one or another gaining ascendancy, depending often on the prevailing attitudes about drugs, politics, young people, and a number of other factors.

What prevention existed prior to the 1960s often involved overblown claims as to the toxicity of illegal drugs. This was often called the "Reefer Madness" approach, after the movie of that name, which depicted the moral and physical disintegration of anyone who so much as sniffed a marijuana "reefer."

The reefer madness approach appears to succeed in situations where there is no actual knowledge of or experience with drugs in the population to which the prevention effort is directed. So long as illegal psychoactive drugs were confined to the ghetto and not a part of general middle-class experience, all the claims as to their dangers were tacitly accepted. In the late 1950s and early 1960s, however, this population began experimenting with marijuana. The emphasis on marijuana and other drug prevention had been on the hypothetical immediate dire moral consequences of use. When these consequences did not occur immediately, the young people who were using marijuana concluded that they had been lied to, and if they had been lied to about marijuana, they were probably being lied to about other drugs as well. Marijuana is a very dangerous drug, but its adverse effects are both subtle and long-term, not the immediately discernible. Prevention experts who rely on scare stories of immediate consequences have forgotten, or perhaps never knew, that the main reason drugs are appealing to young people is that they deliver exactly the positive results that drug experimenters are searching for, at least on the short-term. Very few adolescents look beyond the short-term.

Current versions of "scare tactic" prevention may involve a medical rather than moral approach. Often disputed research results are stated as incontrovertible evidence that this or that drug causes "permanent brain damage" or other irreversible disabilities. There are, of course, highly dangerous and even potentially fatal long-term effects to drug use: AIDS and hepatitis contagion from dirty needles; carcinogenic effects from tobacco; brain, liver, and other internal disease and deterioration from alcohol, and long-term drug-induced psychopathology from pencyclidine, to name only a few. These and other threats need to be researched as thoroughly as possible, and steps taken to inform the public of the risks involved in their use. (The authors think this approach is being very effective in decreasing the levels of tobacco smoking and becoming more effective in dealing with the toxicity and addiction potential of cocaine, but more needs to be done, particularly by physicians, to reach young people, especially those on the fringes of society.)

Overblown claims of permanent damage from even experimental use can backfire into another 60s-style loss of confidence in authority. An even more immediate result is the adverse effect of such claims on those who might seek treatment and successful programs of recovery but decide instead, "What's the use if, according to them, I'm already permanently disabled?"

A better approach is that of teaching the young a realistic assessment of drugs, and their effects. Sound drug education, however, is not enough by itself, and it may even lead to unwarranted experimentation. It should be coupled with help in dealing with the problems that can lead to substance abuse. This includes learning to make sound value judgments, developing a positive self-image and learning to rely on one's inner resources rather than on chemicals in dealing with life's problems.

In calibrating prevention efforts, it is of utmost importance to identify potential addiction as early as possible in its development. Scientists and researchers recognize this and are making strides in learning what may constitute early danger signs and other medical indicators. Given the rapidity with which addiction can develop in the young, pediatricians, family and primary-care physicians and other health professionals who come into contact with teens and pre-teens are in a key position to intervene when signs of possible abuse become apparent.

It is truly the responsibility of every clinician or therapist who comes in contact with adolescent and pre-adolescent populations to become involved in the prevention, identification, assessment, referral, and treatment of alcohol and other drug problems. Although the level and type of involvement may vary somewhat as a function of practice and patient characteristics, physician expertise, and available community resources, no physician can reasonably expect to respond to the physical and psychosocial issues of the adolescents and pre-adolescents without also dealing with alcohol and drugs. In recognition of this basic fact, alcohol, tobacco, and other drug history, screening, and counseling as a component of regular health screening is recommended for 13–18 year olds.[9]

The physician's responsibility to address youth alcohol and drug problems should be considered in light of his or her unique opportunity to address this pressing health problem. Physicians— especially those in primary health-care settings, including social psychiatrists—have opportunities to respond to youth alcohol and drug problems that are not generally available to other profes-sionals who work closely with youth (e.g., teachers and clergy).

The health-care system offers access to large numbers of youth. Surveys conducted by the National Center for Health Statistics reveal that approximately 73% of all American youth (ages 5–24 years) see a doctor at least annually and approxi-mately 50% have seen a doctor within the last 6 months. Although variation is evident as a function of socioeconomic status (SES), race, sex, and general health status, a majority of youth are coming into regular contact with the health-care delivery system. It may be argued that, after the public schools, health-care systems pro-vide the single greatest source of access to the youthful target population. However, unlike the schools, where substance involved youth may be less likely to be reached, substance involved youth are more likely to have contact with the primary health care setting than their non-using counterparts.[10] National survey data[11] reveal that for all reasons for health-care utilization (physical examination, traumatic injury, physical illness or symptom, and emotional and psychological problems), utilization rates are higher for adolescent substance users than for non-users. Moreover, utilization appears to increase as a function of level of substance involvement.

Equally important, the interaction between physician and patient is individualized. It is becoming increasingly clear that an etiologic model applicable to one type of individual may fail to adequately explain the substance-related behavior of another. Thus, the same approach targeted at different youth—different teens in the same community, different students in the same classroom, even different siblings in the same family—will necessarily be of limited efficacy unless the intervention can be tailored to the individual. As Goodstadt[12] notes, "no single strategy is likely to be effective for all drugs and all stages of drug use ... strategies must be tailored to the characteristics of the user, the drug, and the use." This statement is in keeping with the American Society of Addiction Medicine (ASAM) concept of diagnosis-driven treatment. In the health-care system, individualized care, although not always realized in practice is nevertheless a guiding principle.

In addition, physicians possess a unique set of skills and attributes directly relevant to youth alcohol and drug abuse issues. All physicians have had experience in interacting with youth during times of stress or concerning issues of sensitive nature. In many cases, the physician has a long-standing relationship with his or her patient population, providing a unique perspective from which to view physical, emotional, or social changes that may constitute early indications of an emerging alcohol and drug abuse problem.

Finally, physicians who are knowledgeable about substance abuse can be an invaluable resource to other sectors of the community and the nation (parents, schools, policy makers) by serving as informational resources, as a source of referral information, and as credible communicators to and educators of other professionals and lay persons. Moreover, the individual physician and medical/professional organizations have a great deal of influence on health and social policies. Thus, physicians can serve as advocates for legislation, regulation, and policies that reflect scientifically sound and ethically responsible responses to adolescent alcohol and other drug problems.

The Physician's Role as a Practitioner Treating Adolescents and Pre-Adolescents

The physician's primary role (at least in terms of time commitment) in addressing adolescent alcohol and other drug problems is as a clinical practitioner. Virtually every adolescent will experiment with alcohol or other drugs, and a significant minority will progress to heavy or frequent use or will experience substance-related problems such as accidental injury, school and family disruptions, and so on. Thus, there is no adolescent patient for whom alcohol and other drug issues should not be addressed at some level.

Consideration of the physician/adolescent relationship must begin with a reminder that almost all substance use (including alcohol use) is illegal for adolescents. Perhaps more importantly, the majority of young people, including alcohol and other drug users, disapprove of use and realize it is risky. Especially in today's atmosphere of heightened public concern over adolescent alcohol and other drug use, this area is likely to be sensitive for most adolescents, and probably more so than for the adult patient.

In general, physicians who relate well to the adolescent are those who are emphatic, non-judgmental, supportive, and trustworthy; those who relate less well are sanctimonious, authoritarian, condemning, and moralizing. However, the physician can and should express opinions, take positions on issues, make judgments, and use his or her authority when it is in the best interest of the adolescent patient to do so. This may be especially the case in dealing with alcohol and other drugs, where the adolescent is often exposed to a variety of mixed and conflicting messages from parents, peers, and the mass media.

Physician–Patient Relationship

As with any other patient, the relationship between physician and adolescent must be characterized by privacy, confidentiality, and obligation to the patient. These three characteristics of the adolescent–physician relationship may sometimes seem to be in conflict with obligations to the child's parent, but in the absence of a private and confidential atmosphere, the physician will usually be unable to elicit needed information concerning which (if any) substances the adolescent is using, at what dosages and with what frequency, and in what situations. In the absence of this basic information, the physician cannot effectively deal with adolescent substance-related problems.

Most adolescents will provide an accurate description of drug use and associated psychosocial functioning when questioned in an appropriate (i.e., private and confidential) setting. An exception to the general willingness of adolescents to share information concerning alcohol and other drug use is to be expected in the heavily alcohol- or drug-involved adolescent. As has been repeatedly documented for adults, maintenance of heavy substance use often involves the development of skills in deception (including self-deception). Here, the physician's relationship to the adolescent may become one of detective, attempting to reconcile information from parents or school staff, or the physician's own observations when contradictory information is provided by the adolescent patient. Direct confrontation or toxicological screening, although potentially damaging to the immediate relationship, may be in the best interest of the patient.

It is important to note that many of the settings in which adolescents (and adults) receive primary health care (e.g., HMOs, hospital clinics) often do not afford the physician an opportunity to build up a relationship with patients over repeat visits. On the one hand, the anonymity intrinsically afforded by such short-term contact may aid the physician in establishing an atmosphere in which information concerning sensitive behavior such as substance use can be shared by the adolescent. On the other hand, lack of any personal history with the patient makes it all the more important that the physician specifically articulate the ground rules of the interaction.

In order to function effectively as a clinician in addressing adolescent alcohol and other drug problems, the physician must understand his/her relationship to the continuum of substance abuse services. These services include not only in-patient and out-patient drug treatment programs and abstinence-based peer programs (e.g., Alcoholics Anonymous, Narcotics Anonymous, etc.), but also programs to address the range of other problems that substance abusing adolescents experience (e.g., family, educational, mental health) and the range of settings other than the physician's office where substance-involved adolescents may be identified (e.g., schools, courts, human service agencies, places of youth employment).

All physicians should minimally serve as "gate-keepers," identifying and referring troubled adolescents. This role requires a working knowledge of available programs, their inclusionary and exclusionary criteria, and the type and quality of services provided. For the physician who is willing and able to become more involved in adolescent substance abuse treatment—either as a case manager or as the primary agent of treatment—ongoing professional relationships with community programs are essential to ensuring substance-involved youth receive an integrated and complete program of treatment and aftercare. Moreover, such physicians can, themselves, become points of referral for other "gate-keepers" (e.g., schools).

Some physicians may be uncomfortable with or mistrust the competence of paraprofessionals and nonprofessionals. The substance abuse treatment field has long relied on such individuals, in part because of the medical profession's historical reluctance to become involved in the treatment of substance abusers. To the extent that such biases exist, the physician concerned with adolescent substance use and related problems must overcome them, and strive to work as a team member with staff in the broad range of community agencies concerned with adolescent psychosocial problems.

Screening and Intervention

Screening for substance abuse in the pediatric population should begin at the prenatal visit and extend through adolescence.[13,14] A rule of thumb in addiction treatment is that the earlier the problem can be identified and the client brought into treatment, the better the prognosis for recovery. It is better, for example, to identify and treat an alcoholic before organ damage, such as liver disease, sets in. However, the earlier the intervention, the more likely the individual is to have denial. With chemically dependent adolescents, the need for early detection is even more acute than it is with adults. The course from beginning of use to full addiction is much more rapid in adolescents than it is in adults, so every month, every day, counts for a great deal.

A physician or other health professional who is already in contact with an adolescent in general, pediatric or family practice is in a good position to recognize chemical dependency clients at an early stage if the therapist is sensitive to changes in behavior that are characteristic to chemical dependency.

The identification and diagnosis of alcohol and other drug problems among adolescent populations poses a number of conceptual and practical difficulties. Chief among these is the lack of consistently applied definitions of abuse and dependence in adolescents. The nosology of adolescent alcohol and other drug-related problems is underdeveloped, and diagnostic criteria applied to adults are of questionable relevance to adolescent populations. (Note: For that reason, the diagnostic criteria for adolescents developed by the American Society on Addiction Medicine is appended to the end of this chapter.)

A second difficulty is the growing attractiveness of chemical dependency treatment, and the reduced stigma attached to the chemical dependency label. Adolescents, or their parents, may seek a diagnosis of chemical dependency in situations where chemical involvement may not be the primary difficulty. Parents may prefer to believe that their child is chemically dependent, rather than mentally disturbed, delinquent, or facing chaotic or unwholesome family circumstances. As adolescent chemical dependency treatment facilities become the programs of first choice rather than of last resort, the need to sort out target problems and make appropriate referral decisions will increase.

There is also growing concern about the ethics and marketing techniques of treatment providers and fear that adolescents are inappropriately referred for drug treatment. Moreover, the Juvenile Justice and Delinquency Prevention Act of 1974, which prohibits the incarceration of status offenders, has led to the placement of these adolescents in chemical dependency treatment centers even when such placement is not appropriate.[15] Further, adolescents may mature out of their drug use patterns without formal intervention or treatment. Thus, it is necessary to exercise caution in assigning diagnostic labels that represent a chronic, progressive disease for which lifetime abstinence is the foundation of treatment of choice.

A final difficulty is that many of the alcohol and other drug problems experienced by adolescents do not fit traditional notions of "abuse" or "dependence." An adolescent who is an episodic user of alcohol, but whose use patterns place him or her at high risk of accidental injury is clearly in need of attention from the physician. Moreover, many adolescents who do not, themselves, use alcohol or other drugs may be put at risk by their association with users. Riding with intoxicated drivers appears to be a common occurrence among adolescents, and this behavior may put non-drug using adolescents at as much risk of injury as their drug-using counterparts. Another important risk is the relation of unsafe sex to intoxication, producing a high-risk for AIDS and other sexually transmitted diseases.

Cognizant of the above considerations, and absent standard diagnostic criteria for adolescent alcohol and other drug abuse and dependence, the task of the practitioner is to assess as fully as possible the patient's level of substance-related risk and to formulate a plan of action that is responsive to and consistent with that assessment.

An individual adolescent's substance-related risk will vary as a function of the type of substance used, the frequency and quantity of use, the settings where use takes place, and the route of administration. Risk will also vary as a function of biological and intrapsychic differences, and factors in the individual's family, school, and peer environments. An assessment of risk may involve any or all of the following: (1) screening instruments; (2) alcohol and other drug history; (3) assessment of signs and symptoms; (4) physical examination; (5) psychological test; and (6) laboratory tests.

Screening Instruments

It has been argued that the time constraints of the health-care setting dictate the need for a simple, efficient mechanism by which to screen adolescents for potential substance abuse problems. Advocates of this position cite evidence that rates of identification of adolescent substance abuse problems in health settings is low, and that practitioners underestimate the prevalence of such problems in their patient populations. Moreover, it is argued that adolescents may be reluctant to share sensitive information, and may be more willing to do so through a pre-visit questionnaire than through a face-to-face interview with the physician.[9]

There is little disagreement that such questionnaires can be a useful adjunct to patient interviews and other assessment strategies. However, the use of such instruments to identify adolescents in need of further assessment (and, conversely to identify those who do not need further assessment) is inappropriate for two reasons. First, the reliability and validity of most available adolescent screening tools has not been well established, and even the best screening tools will misclassify large numbers of adolescents. Second, a discussion of alcohol and other drug issues is required for all adolescents, even those who are not current users.

The therapist who chooses to use screening questionnaires in his or her practice should view the screening tool as a starting point for discussion. Thus, for example, the physician can go over the questionnaire items or summary scores with the patient, probing for the reasons underlying the patient's responses. Questionnaire responses from the current visit might also be compared by physician and patient to questionnaire responses from previous visits in order to look for and confront inconsistencies, and to gain insight into the ways in which the patient's alcohol and other drug-related behavior is evolving.

Used as a starting point for discussion, screening questionnaires will facilitate the development of a comprehensive understanding of the substance-related issues faced by the adolescent patient. However, physicians who use screening questionnaires as a "short-cut" substitute for a candid and confidential discussion of alcohol and other drug use are not fulfilling their responsibilities to their adolescent patients.

Alcohol and Other Drug History

The alcohol and other drug history should accomplish two major goals. First, it should provide a complete picture of which, if any, substances the patient is using, the quantity and frequency of use, and the settings for use. Second, it should provide insight into any life areas in which the patient is experiencing difficulties. These difficulties may be sequelae of alcohol and other drug use or they may be predictive of future alcohol and other drug problems.

There exist no standardized guidelines for the variables to be assessed in an adolescent alcohol and other drug history.

However, based on current understandings of the etiology and sequelae of adolescent alcohol and other drug use, nine areas of inquiry can be identified: (1) overall adjustment, (2) family history, including past and current use patterns of family members, (3) use patterns of peers and close friends, (4) attitudes toward use, (5) current functioning in family, (6) current functioning in school, (7) social activities and peer relations, (8) juvenile justice involvement, and (9) treatment and current use patterns.

■ ISSUES TO ADDRESS IN AN ADOLESCENT ALCOHOL AND OTHER DRUG HISTORY

Overall Adjustment:

1. What stresses are currently being experienced? How well is the patient coping with these stresses?
2. Is the patient depressed, bored, or lonely?
3. Does the patient feel alienated?
4. Does the patient have goals or plans for the future?

Family History and Use Patterns:

1. Do parents smoke, drink, or use other drugs? To what extent?
2. Do siblings smoke, drink, or use other drugs? To what extent?
3. Has a parent or sibling received treatment for chemical dependency?
4. Does the patient believe that a parent or sibling has an alcohol or other drug problem?
5. Would parents approve of use by the patient?

Use Patterns of Peers and Close Friends:

1. Do friends smoke, drink, or use other drugs? To what extent?
2. Do friends approve of use?
3. Do friends have ready access to alcohol and other drugs?
4. Do friends drive after using alcohol or other drugs? Is the patient a passenger with these friends?

Attitudes Toward Use:

1. Does the patient approve of tobacco, alcohol, or other drug use for someone his/her age? Under what circumstances?
2. Would the patient like to try tobacco, alcohol, or other drugs?

Family Functioning:

1. Do the patient's parents generally know where the patient is and what he/she is doing? Has the patient ever run away from home?
2. Does that patient feel that he/she is valued by family members?
3. How much time does the patient spend with his/her parents?
4. Do the patients parents set rules? Enforce rules consistently?
5. Do the patient's parents approve of his/her friends?
6. Have the patient's parents discussed rules and expectations concerning alcohol and other drug use? Concerning driving after drinking?
7. Has the patient been sexually or physically abused?

School Functioning:

1. Has the patient been making passing marks?
2. Does the patient like school? Feel safe and welcome at school? Believe his/her teachers care about him/her?
3. Has the patient been truant? Repeatedly tardy?
4. Has the patient been in trouble at school?
5. Does the patient fight with other students?
6. Does the patient intend to complete high school? Does he/she plan to go to college?

Social Activities and Peer Relations:

1. Does the patient participate in *adult supervised* recreation (teams, clubs, church groups)?
2. Does the patient attend parties where alcohol and other drugs are available? Where drinking games are played?
3. How often does the patient go out with friends on school nights?

4. Does the patient have at least one close, confidential relationship?
5. Does the patient feel comfortable relating to peers?
6. Have the patient's friends or peer group changed recently?
7. Are many of the patient's friends at least two years older than the patient?

Juvenile Justice Involvement:

1. Has the patient ever been arrested for driving while intoxicated?
2. Has the patient had any other contacts with law enforcement or the courts?

Current Use Patterns:

1. How many times per week/month does the patient drink alcoholic beverages? How many times per week/month does the patient drink to intoxication?
2. How much does the patient typically drink?
3. Has the patient ever experienced a black-out after drinking?
4. Does the patient smoke cigarettes or use smokeless tobacco? How often?
5. Does the patient use other drugs (marijuana, cocaine, crack, stimulants, PCP, inhalants, hallucinogens, opiates, steroids)? How often? With which mode(s) of ingestion/administration?
6. In what settings does the patient use alcohol and other drugs (at parties, at school, at home, in friends' homes, alone)?
7. Does the patient ever drive after or while using alcohol or other drugs? Does the patient use safety belts?
8. Has the patient's use been increasing (more substance or more potent substances)?
9. Has the patient ever tried to cut down on use? With what result?

Clearly, not all of the issues listed above need be addressed with all adolescents. For example, many of the variables will not be addressed with patients who have not yet experimented with alcohol or other drugs. Also, the variables need not be addressed in any particular order. In general, the physician will begin with less threatening topics, such as attitudes towards use, or use by peers, and move to progressively more threatening topics such as use by family members and use by the patient.

A complete alcohol and other drug history is time consuming, especially if the physician covers all the topics listed above. Unfortunately, there are no simple short-cuts. Ultimately, the physician must rely on his or her clinical judgment to determine whether a particular avenue of inquiry (such as family adjustment or school performance) is likely to yield useful information. At the very least, the physician should gather complete information on use patterns by the patient and his or her immediate family. Without this basic information, it is not possible to begin to address the multiple types and levels of alcohol and other drug problems adolescent patients experience.

Perhaps the most important factor in obtaining an accurate alcohol and other drug history is the relationship of the physician to the patient. The physician must communicate his/her interest in the patient's experience with alcohol and other drugs as a health issue, the confidentiality of the doctor/patient interaction, the acceptability of sharing information concerning alcohol and other drug use, and the willingness of the physician to serve as an informational and helping resource.

It is important to note that current understanding of both the precursors of and sequelae to alcohol and other drug use is imperfect. Not all adolescent alcohol and other drug users experience life disruptions, and not all adolescents who exhibit risk factors for alcohol and other drug use actually go on to become users. As has been repeatedly emphasized, all adolescent users of alcohol and other drugs are at increased risk. The goal of the alcohol and drug history is to establish the extent of risk, and to aid in planning an appropriate response.

Two rules of thumb may be applied in evaluating the significance of findings from the alcohol and other drug history:

1. The greater the quantity, frequency, and variety of substance use the more likely it is that problems will occur.

2. The greater the number of risk factors with which an individual adolescent must cope, the greater the probability of alcohol and other drug problems.

The practitioner can use the alcohol and other drug history in three ways. First, the adolescent's responses to questions in the alcohol and other drug history should form the basis for in-office counseling and guidance about specific risk behaviors. For example, adolescents who report driving after drinking, or riding with intoxicated drivers should be counseled about the risk associated with these behaviors and should be provided with suggestions of strategies to avoid them, such as avoiding parties where alcohol is served, calling parents for a ride, or using public transportation. *Note*: it is important for adolescents to find a social situation in which alcohol and other drugs are not used, and for them to develop a supportive, substance-free peer group.

Second, the practitioner should be alert to changes in functioning which may be indicative of emerging alcohol or other drug problems. These would include changes in any of the life domains included in the list, i.e., overall adjustment, family, school, social activities and peer relations, or escalation in quantity, frequency, or diversity of substance use patterns.

Finally, the practitioner should be alert to indications that an alcohol or other drug problem has reached the point where an in-depth, diagnostic assessment and/or referral for treatment may be required. This is the most difficult assessment to make based on the alcohol and other drug history. It is rare that an alcohol or other drug problem requiring intensive intervention will be uncovered during routine history taking, in part because the heavily substance-involved adolescent may be uncooperative or may deny that such a problem exists. Rather, the practitioner must make a clinical judgment based upon the overall pattern of responses obtained from the adolescent and determine whether a more in-depth assessment, either by the physician or through a referral, is indicated. Tools for in-depth assessments of substance involved adolescents are discussed later in this section.

Presenting Complaints That May Be Related to Substance Abuse

Most adolescent alcohol and other drug users are asymptomatic. Unless the adolescent patient is intoxicated at the time of contact with the physician, there will generally be little obvious evidence of an alcohol or other drug problem. However, there are at least six presenting complaints that should raise the physician's index of suspicion and occasion an in-depth assessment of alcohol or other drug involvement as part of treatment planning. These are: (1) traumatic injury, (2) suicide attempts, (3) depression, (4) school failure, (5) family disruptions, and (6) delinquency or other anti-social behavior problems. In each case, the correlation between these problems and substance abuse is strong.

■ PHYSICAL EXAMINATION

The physical examination provides an excellent opportunity to engage the adolescent in conversation, and may be used to initiate the substance abuse history. However, unless an adolescent patient is intoxicated at the time of an office or emergency room visit, the results of the physical examination of all but the most heavily substance involved adolescents will generally be un-remarkable. Classic adult markers of chronic substance abuse, such as cirrhosis of the liver, are virtually unknown in adolescents. Thus, the physical examination itself will generally be of limited utility in the identification and diagnosis of adolescent substance use and abuse.

Symptoms as seen in adolescents with the disease of chemical dependence are similar to those seen in adults; however, because of their age and lack of personality development and maturity, these symptoms may become exacerbated and tele-scope (intensify and shorten) the progression of the disease. In addition, lack of job skills or income along with a tendency to run away can lead teenagers into illegal activities or to suicide.

■ SIGNS AND SYMPTOMS OF CHEMICAL DEPENDENCE IN ADOLESCENTS

1. For addicted adolescents, life becomes centered around alcohol and drugs. Peer groups change dramatically. Friends are now almost exclusively alcohol and drug users.
2. At this stage, adolescents are drinking and using to "maintain"; they are not drinking for euphoria but for freedom from the pain and the hurt they are almost continually experiencing.
3. Repeated attempts to stay stopped are made, yet such attempts are unsuccessful. They may stop for 2 or 3 days or 2 or 3 weeks or months, but subsequently resume use. This ability to stop chemical use for a limited period of time leads adolescents to mistakenly believe that they can control their chemical use.
4. Physical deterioration may begin to occur in either appearance and/or physical health. Weight loss, in addition to dental, gum and complexion problems, also tends to occur during the course of the disease, as well as a general lethargy translated as being "burned out" or "spaced out." There may also be a deterioration in personal hygiene or clothing. There may be serious physical withdrawal symptoms when one tries to stop using drugs; and GI problems, nervous problems, cardiac, or liver problems may result.
5. Hiding and lying about drug use is common. There is no reason to hide one's use, or to lie about it, if there is no problem.
6. Using drugs and alcohol alone occurs. At this stage, use is no longer simply a matter of peer acceptance or peer affiliation.
7. Denial is one of the major symptoms of the disease. It is manifested by an altered perception of reality, and by repression of pain that one experiences. Two "dragons of denial" exist: the dragon of deceit and the dragon of self-deception. The dragons tell addicts that they can control use by themselves and that they can stop at any time.
8. Increased feelings of aloneness and isolation occur. Every alcoholic and drug addict who continues to use chemicals

eventually will find himself or herself in the center of the target syndrome. It is a disease of "de-peoplization." The chemically dependent adolescent essentially peels people away just as one would peel off the layers of an onion, or the circles of a target, until one gets to the "bulls-eye." First, church activities go, then community activities, then jobs, then school, then peers, then friends, then members of the distant family, and finally members of the immediate family. At last, the chemically dependent adolescent is completely alone, truly isolated and de-peoplized at the center of the target, with nothing left but the chemical.

9. Concern is expressed by parents, teachers, and significant others, even peers. (You know you are in trouble when using buddies and peers become concerned about your behavior or drug use.)

10. Guarding one's supply becomes important. In other words, one always manages to have "some on hand, just in case."

11. Frequent visits to physicians, emergency rooms, or continued need for medications may occur. Psychosomatic complaints may be present, as well as an increased number of accidents and traumas (particularly burns and falls).

12. Gradually, a loss of self-esteem occurs, with an increase in denial and the accompanying anger and depression. Certainly, these are psychiatric symptoms, but symptoms secondary to the disease of chemical dependence, not primary psychopathology. When the drugs are removed, and a period of chemical abstinence occurs, the psychiatric manifestations generally disappear.

13. Serious family conflicts, with increasing fragmentation, disorganization, and eventual chaos may occur. Confrontation within the family can be seen, with fighting among brothers and sisters, running-away behavior, and isolation from family activities.

14. All of the above characteristics are examples of manifestations of the chief symptom of the disease—*Loss of Control. When loss of control occurs, then chemical use persists despite consequences suffered.*

During the abusing stage, the behavior controls the chemicals. Once the biochemical-genetic wall is crossed, the chemicals control the behavior. The addict can no longer guarantee his or her behavior when using chemicals. Abuse is a cortical (rational and logical) process; addiction acts as an instinctual urge does. Addiction is controlled by a deeper, more primitive (i.e., lower) center of the brain. The addict's compulsion to use the chemical arises from the primitive instinctual centers or the Hypothalamic Instinctual Control Center (HICC). The HICC is the site where most instinctual impulses arise and is also the area of the brain where deficiencies in central neurotransmitters, i.e., naturally occurring brain chemicals, occur that may lead to addiction. These neurotransmitters are responsible for behavior and feelings. Consequently, the theory is that chemically dependent individuals are actually addicted to the feeling the drug causes, not the actual drug itself. Therefore, one's drug of choice is determined by the natural feeling the triggered neurotransmitter produces.

Guidelines for Adolescent Interviewing Procedure

The following guidelines, interview and parent information guides are based on materials developed by George C. Comerci for his article "Office Assessment and Brief Intervention with the Adolescent Suspected of Substance Abuse" in *Principles of Addiction Medicine.*[16]

Approach:

1. Begin by discussing more general life-style questions, including the following topic areas: home/family relations, functioning at school, peer relationships, leisure activities, employment, and self-perception.
2. Ask about dietary patterns.
3. Proceed to questions about prescribed medications.
4. Ask about over-the-counter medications.
5. Inquire about cigarettes and smokeless tobacco use.

6. Learn about the use of alcohol.
7. Question the adolescent about the use of marijuana.
8. Finally, ask about the use of any illicit drug.

Rationale:

1. Allow time to develop or renew the patient–physician relationship.
2. Provide a basis (through general psycho-social information) for determining the patient's risk for a harmful environment.
3. Start with the least threatening questions.
4. Move to increasingly sensitive substances.
5. This order of questioning provides a natural order of progression, moving from the socially accepted to the socially tolerated to the socially disapproved to the overtly illegal.

Essentials for a Structured Interview:

- What drugs are used?
- How frequently is each drug used?
- At what age did the patient begin using each drug?
- What is the setting in which each drug is used?
- What has been the level of intoxication with each drug (including blackout spells and periods of amnesia)?
- Has use of drug(s) resulted in involvement with the police or arrest?
- Has use of drug(s) put the patient in high-risk situations?
- Has use of drug(s) caused school absences or deterioration of school grades?
- Has use of drug(s) affected relationships with family or friends or affected a romantic relationship?

Information from Parents:

- Do family members, including parents, have an alcohol or other drug problem?
- Is there a family history of depression (especially bipolar affective disorder), suicide or suicide attempt, or other psychiatric illness?

- What changes have the parents noted in your child's mood, affect, behavior or dress?
- Has there been lying to cover up for absences from home or school, for missing personal or family belongings, or for "no good reason at all?"
- Have the child's personal belongings or family possessions or money been missing?
- Has the child's manner of dress or personal hygiene changed?
- Have drug paraphernalia been found in the child's possession or in the home?
- Has there been stealing, shoplifting, or encounters with the police?
- Has there been deterioration in the child's school performance, frequent truancy, or conflict with coaches or teachers?
- Has the child been physically abusive to you or your spouse?
- Has the child tried to introduce drugs or alcohol to any of your other children?
- Has the child talked about suicide or running away?

Assessment and Referral

A fundamental goal of each evaluation is that the physician be able to determine both whether the patient is using drugs and, if so, whether that use is experimental and casual, or problematic. It is also important that the physician determine the stage of drug use or abuse that the patient is in. A structured interview goes a long way in improving the efficiency of the evaluation and lessens the amount of time needed for data collection. Such an interview should have definite objectives and provide the physician with specific questions to ask, while appearing to be spontaneous and flexible. And it should be targeted toward gathering certain important information.

Depression and other psychiatric diagnoses should be considered. A history of physical or sexual abuse, or both, may be relevant. Information from parents is often critical.

The limitations on the use of questionnaires underscore the need for trust to be established and maintained and for privacy and confidentiality to be ensured. The adolescent and young adult are aware that if they confide in the physician regarding substantial drug abuse, such information will be used to intervene. Most persons involved in abuse of chemicals are not interested in changing their behavior, and lying in order to avoid disclosure is not unusual.

In the final analysis, in the case of data collection for the identification of substance abuse and chemical dependence, valid information is more likely to result from a skilled interview than from a perfectly structured and designed questionnaire. Whatever method is used, accurate and honest responses by the adolescent or young adult are going to depend, in large part, on the degree to which trust is established and on the extent to which the patient perceives the physician as a caring, helpful, and knowledgeable adult. For the physician who chooses to use questionnaires as a tool for more efficient data collection, a number of screening and assessment instruments are available.

■ LABORATORY ASSESSMENT

The use of urine or other body fluid testing to identify adolescents who are abusing drugs is an attractive alternative to the time-consuming interview and physical examination. The accuracy of modern testing methods notwithstanding, there are many reasons, both ethical and practical, however, why this approach remains controversial. There are special indications for laboratory testing. Comerci[16] is of the opinion that testing is probably justified only when (1) it is requested by a parent, (2) in order to save time, (3) in cases in which one does not trust the veracity of the adolescent, or (4) for the reason that it is part of a medical work-up, such as testing for tuberculosis.

Trust is necessary for a therapeutic alliance to be established with the adolescent. Effective ways to prevent a trusting relation-

ship from developing are to test without the young person's knowledge, to test in spite of the adolescent's objections, or to test on
parent demand. However, an out of control adolescent or an adolescent who shows evidence of serious dysfunction is an exception
to the general rule. There is no problem in testing patients who provide voluntary consent but it is most unlikely that the substance-
abusing adolescent will give consent for a test that may very well
show that he or she is lying.

■ ASSESSMENT AND EVALUATION

The assessment of substance-related problems in adolescents can
sometimes be facilitated by the use of in-depth psychological
tests. Such tests have the advantage of increased objectivity
when compared to clinical interviews. They may also provide specific scoring criteria for establishing a diagnosis and/or normative
data against which the responses of the adolescent patient may
be compared.

Psychological tests relevant to the assessment of adolescent
substance abuse may be categorized into three major types:
(1) psychiatric interview protocols, (2) substance use/abuse
assessments, and (3) comprehensive assessment batteries.

Psychiatric Interview Protocols

Psychiatric interview protocols are designed to yield diagnoses for
a variety of mental disorders including substance-related disorders. In general, these interview protocols rely on diagnostic criteria established by the *Diagnostic and Statistical Manual, Fourth
Edition* (DSM-IV) of the American Psychiatric Association. Four
widely used psychiatric interview protocols are:

- The Diagnostic Interview Schedule for Children (DISC).
- The children's version of the Schedule for Affective
  Disorders and Schizophrenia (Kiddie-SADS).

- The National Institute on Mental Health Diagnostic Interview Schedule for Children.
- The Child Assessment Schedule.

A major advantage of these interview schedules is the breadth of information they provide. Because substance abuse often co-occurs with other mental disorders (the dual diagnosis adolescent), the availability of diagnoses in a wide range of disorders can facilitate treatment planning.

The administration of psychiatric interview schedules usually requires a trained interviewer. Thus, these schedules will generally be of limited use in office practice and will usually require a referral to a practitioner trained in their use and interpretation.

Substance Use/Abuse Assessments

Most assessments specifically designed for adolescent substance use/abuse are screening tools of the type discussed earlier. One exception is the *Personal Experience Inventory* (PEI) developed by the Chemical Dependency Adolescent Projects.[17]

The PEI is a two-part paper-and-pencil assessment which yields a profile of substance abuse problem severity, an assessment of a variety of substance-related psychosocial variables, and a measure of invalid responding.

Part I (Problem Severity Scales) includes 10 scales which measure settings of use, effects from use, consequences of use, pre-occupation with use, and loss of control. Part I also contains three scales which help determine the validity of the patient's responses.

Part II of the PEI (Psychosocial Scales) contains 8 scales which measure personal adjustment problems, such as negative self-image, social isolation, aggressiveness, and spiritual isolation; and 4 scales that measure environmental risk factors, i.e., substance use by peers, substance use by siblings, family pathology, and family conflict.

Completion by the patient of both sections of the PEI takes about 45 minutes to 1 hour. Research studies of the PEI have established the reliability and validity of the scales, and the scales have compared favorably to both clinical diagnoses and scores from other psychological batteries.

■ COMPREHENSIVE ASSESSMENT BATTERIES

Successful treatment planning for adolescent patients will likely involve more than simply matching clients to treatments based on the severity of substance involvement. Drug use patterns and history are clearly related to treatment outcomes. However, adolescent drug abuse is associated with a variety of problems in other life domains which also appear to be correlated with overall treatment success. These include psychiatric problems, criminality, educational difficulties and dropping out, family problems including abuse and victimization, and lack of positive involvement in productive roles. Accordingly, the most successful treatment planning for adolescent substance abusers will need to address a wide variety of problem areas and services related to these areas.

In 1987, the National Institute on Drug Abuse (NIDA) launched an ambitious, multi-year project to develop a comprehensive adolescent assessment and referral system (AARS) that would screen and assess adolescents suspected of substance-related problems in 10 life domains: (1) substance use/abuse, (2) physical health status, (3) mental health status, (4) family relationships, (5) peer relations, (6) educational status, (7) vocational status, (8) social skills, (9) leisure and recreation, and (10) aggressive behavior/delinquency.[17]

The AARS consists of a paper-and-pencil screening tool to identify domains in which further assessment is indicated, clinically validated, in-depth assessments in each of the 10 domains, and a guide for making referrals to treatment based on assessment results. The AARS subsumes some of the diagnostic assessments discussed earlier. For example, the PEI is used as the in-depth assessment instrument for the substance use/abuse domain and the DISC is used as the in-depth assessment in the mental health status domain.

■ POSITIVE OUTCOME

Early detection and intervention for the substance-abusing adolescent are necessary if the progress of the disorder, its detrimental effect on normal development and its contribution to death and morbidity are to be prevented. The leading causes of death among adolescents and young adults are accidents, homicides and suicides, a significant number of which are associated with alcohol and other drug use. The effectiveness of our interventions and treatment programs for substance abuse is uncertain. Many physicians are skeptical of the claims of success by addiction specialists and programs, and they therefore fail to intervene or refer. Difficulties in determining outcome have to do with differences among the adolescents being referred for treatment, proper matching of treatment to a given adolescent's needs, different markers of success (e.g., total drug abstinence, return to successful life functioning, controlled use), differences between short- and long-term follow-up outcomes, differences between the assessment instruments used for adolescents and those used for adults and differences in the problem of substance abuse between adolescents and adults. Success rates vary from 15% to 45%, depending on whether short- or long-term outcome is being assessed. For juvenile drug abusers, there is a steady improvement over a 7-year period. However, the degree to which that improvement is attributable to maturational gains (the "maturing out process") as opposed to treatment is not known.

Until further research has been conducted to document treatment success, primary-care clinicians must realize that it is not yet possible to know which adolescents are most amenable to help; they will have to assume that some treatment, even if imperfect, is better than none at all.

■ NEGATIVE CONSEQUENCES OF MISSED DIAGNOSES AND NON-INTERVENTION

The stages of substance use and abuse begin with the potential for and vulnerability to substance abuse, and they extend through experimentation, drug seeking, preoccupation with drugs, and finally physical and psychological chemical dependence. The concept of "gateway drugs" is probably an erroneous one; the belief that one drug necessarily or inevitably leads to the use of "harder" drugs is incomplete if not invalid. Rather, the use of illicit drugs is more dependent on antecedents present at all stages, and certain peer and parental influences are present throughout the continuum of use and abuse. As important is the observation that there is a pattern of lessening use as an adolescent moves through young adulthood. It appears that involvement with drugs and alcohol begins during early to mid-adolescence, reaches a peak in late adolescence and young adulthood, and then decreases (except for cigarettes) after age 22. These observations of improvement without treatment should not cause the clinician to abandon efforts toward identification and intervention, but rather, should intensify his or her commitment to early intervention. Considering that violent deaths during adolescence and young adulthood are frequently associated with drugs and alcohol, physicians should be aware that intervention provides a reasonable chance of survival for an individual not necessarily doomed to lifelong problems with drugs and their harmful effects. Much will have been accomplished if a physician intervenes early, allowing a patient to survive through this critical "mellowing out" period.

Treatment Referral

Once an assessment has been made and an initial evaluation achieved, the next step may be referral. Can the problem be resolved through office visits and counseling? Is referral to a 12-Step program appropriate? Is referral to a treatment facility called for? If so, what kind? Initial referral is discussed as is referral following relapse into use.

Some adolescents who suffer alcohol and other drug (AOD) problems can be adequately managed in the primary-care setting, depending on the intensity of their AOD involvement and the clinician's level of interest, knowledge and skills. Other patients will require a level and intensity of services best offered in specialized treatment settings.

Therapeutic interventions can be made to correspond to the nature of the patient's alcohol or drug problem if treatment is conceptualized as a series of steps that increase in intensity relative to problem severity.

Thus, using the Levels of Severity that follow this section, low-intensity interventions are used for Levels 1 and 2, while higher intensity treatments are reserved for severity Levels 3–5. This approach needs to be modified in the face of several special considerations. For example, the drug-dependent adolescent who also has serious medical problems usually is best treated on a general medical unit. In such cases, the primary treatment is medical, but support personnel can be enlisted to help carry out detoxification if needed and enhance the patient's receptiveness to long-term rehabilitation.

Patients with serious primary affective disorders should be referred to a psychiatrist. If these patients have active suicidal ideation, they should be treated in a psychiatric facility where appropriate patient safeguards can be provided. After detoxification, any indicated pharmacologic treatment of the affective disorder can be initiated.

Treatment Plan Guidelines

Because some patients who seek assistance for an alcohol or drug-related crisis may be prepared to 'do almost anything" to make matters improve, physicians should consider these guidelines in developing a treatment plan:[18]

1. *Justify your actions.* Because alcohol and drug problems tend to fluctuate naturally in intensity, regardless of the mode of intervention, the physician must constantly justify his actions in terms of benefits vs financial costs, patient and staff time, physical and emotional hazards to the patient, and the trauma of separation from family and friends.

2. *Know the natural course of the disorder.* Development of an adequate treatment plan is possible only if the physician understands the probable course of various patterns of abuse.

3. *Match the treatment approach to the patient's needs.* Select the least costly, least potentially harmful and simplest treatment approach that meets the patient's needs, unless there are good data to justify more complex procedures.

4. *Apply objective diagnostic criteria.* Standard diagnostic criteria should be applied to each patient in order to understand the natural course of his dependence and predict future problems. An individual may be labeled "ill but undiagnosed" or assigned a working diagnosis, but care must be taken to re-evaluate these labels at a later date. In addition, all patients should be evaluated for major pre-existing physical or psychiatric disorders that require specific treatment or affect the prognosis.

5. *Establish realistic goals.* The physician's objectives should be to maximize the patient's chances for recovery, to encourage abstinence in a shorter time than might have been achieved without intervention, to offer good medical care, to help the people close to the patient understand the course of the patient's illness and treatment, and to educate the patient's family so that they can make informed decisions about treatment methods and goals.

6. *Understand the patient's motivations.* It is important to understand the adolescent patient's reasons for entering treatment: adolescents rarely seek treatment. Therefore, given the understanding that the adolescent patient is under duress, does he or she seek long-term abstinence, or is his or her actual goal detoxification or help in meeting a crisis? Or is

there a goal beyond complying with parental demands and wishes?

7. *Make a long-term commitment.* Recovery from alcohol and drug-related problems usually is a long-term process, requiring some counseling and continuation of a therapeutic relationship for at least 12–14 months post-treatment.

8. *Use interpersonal resources.* Part of the treatment effort should be directed to encouraging the patient's family, school and/or employer to understand the patient's problem. With such understanding, these important resources can help the patient achieve recovery and, to some extent, function as "ancillary therapists" in helping to carry out the treatment plan in the home, school or workplace.

9. *Do not take final responsibility for the patient's actions.* In the final analysis, the decision to achieve and maintain abstinence is the patient's responsibility. If the patient initially stops using alcohol or drugs only to please the physician, or his or her parents, he or she will soon find an excuse to become angry and resume abuse.

Above all, the physician should attempt to establish a consistent, continuing relationship with the patient, no matter what course of treatment is selected.

■ OVERCOMING DENIAL

Denial is present in nearly all adolescents who are actively addicted to alcohol or other drugs. This response may be evidenced by one or more of the following mechanisms:

- Conscious lying (one of the least common mechanisms).
- Classic denial (an adaptive coping response to avoid a distressing problem).
- Memory blackout.
- Euphoric recall (the patient remembers only the good times associated with drinking or using drugs).
- Wishful or magical thinking.
- Denial on the part of family and other close persons.

- Ignorance of the nature of addictive disease.
- Toxic effects of the abused substance on information processing and memory.
- Stigma related to the terms "alcoholic" and "addict."
- Fear of the unknown.
- A complex thinking quandary (this consists of genuine confusion on the part of the patient, who knows that something is wrong in his or her life, but who cannot connect the problem with his or her alcohol or other drug abuse).

Denial protects persons with alcohol and drug disorders from conscious awareness of the disease process, and permits them to continue drinking and/or using drugs despite adverse consequences. Society believes that addicts are weak, bad, crazy, stupid, and immoral. The shame arising out of prescribing to these beliefs about addiction creates denial to protect the adolescent addict's ego and sense of self. It is, therefore, the underlying psychological component of the disease process.

■ COMPLIANCE

While most adolescents follow medical advice, many do not. It is not primarily a matter of compliance with the physician's wishes, but rather a question as to why the adolescent does or does not act in his or her own best interest.

What are some of the factors that foster a therapeutic alliance between the physician and the adolescent?

Encouragement of Families to Participate in the Treatment Process

Active participation of the patient's family or significant other helps these important persons understand their role in the patient's continuing recovery. Through such participation, family members learn how to set appropriate limits and how to adopt realistic expectations for the patient in recovery. Family participation also helps family members and significant others address the toll the patient's addiction has had on their own health and emotional well-being. It should be noted, though, that both within and beyond the middle class, adolescent addicts often have no intact family.

Providing Feedback

The physician's objective feedback about the nature and severity of alcohol and drug-related problems can prompt change. Making clear the discrepancy between a patient's present state and the patient's desired state leads to dissatisfaction which becomes a source of motivation. Combining feedback with training in coping skills can further enhance effectiveness.

Setting Goals

Feedback in the absence of a goal appears to be ineffective. Goals and feedback enhance each other as motivational interventions. Feedback about present negative consequences may induce a discrepancy and an intention to change. Progress toward a clear goal then proceeds, influenced and reinforced by continuing feedback regarding the remaining degree of discrepancy.

Maintaining Contact

Some of the most successful motivational interventions are relatively simple, involving continuity of contact between patient and primary physician. For example, patients receiving a personal follow-up letter expressing concern for their welfare and inviting further consultation were found to have a significantly higher self-referral rate for substance abuse treatment. Following a missed appointment, a simple telephone call or a personal letter expressing interest in the patient increase the probability of the patient returning.

■ MAKING EFFECTIVE REFERRALS

In order for the physician to make effective referrals for adolescent patients with alcohol and other drug-related problems, he or she must be aware of and understand the range of services designed for such patients. Moreover, it is important for the physician to become familiar with services available in the local community and must be aware of the practical barriers that may interfere with patient compliance. In addition, he or she must have a working knowledge of the evidence of effectiveness of various programmatic approaches.

■ MATCHING REFERRALS TO PATIENT NEEDS

Effective referrals must be based on a thorough assessment of the patient's problems in all significant life domains and on a familiarity with the patient's general life situation. With this knowledge, the physician is more likely to be able to match referral resources to the patient's most pressing needs. This matching process has two important components: First, the physician must refer to resources that are accessible and practically appropriate for the patient. Second, the physician must refer to resources that match the particular problems of the patient.

The nature and availability of resources to provide help to alcohol and other drug involved adolescents vary greatly from community to community. Depending on a variety of variables, the physician may have the opportunity to choose from a broad range of programs and providers and attempt to closely match services with the adolescents personal characteristics and needs. In other cases, the existing and accessible resources may be quite limited and the physician's task may be less one of trying to find just the right match and more one of tracking down any resources at all.

The first issue that the physician must deal with is accessibility. Financial limitations may be the most serious barrier. Unless families have substantial financial resources or insurance coverage, many programs and providers may not be accessible. Geographic accessibility must also be considered. In some instances, for example an inpatient program, a treatment facility located at some distance from the patient's home community may have advantages in that it removes the adolescent from unhealthy influences. In most cases, however, distances may make family participation difficult.

There are other access issues. Some programs will not accept pregnant patients. Some programs will not accept patients with learning disabilities or a history of aggressive or violent behavior. Some programs require significant participation by parents, which may not be feasible.

The second overall component of making appropriate referrals is matching the services to the patient's needs. One aspect of matching is making sure that all of the patient's major needs are considered. It is generally associated with mental health problems, family problems, and educational and vocational difficulties. Substance abuse rarely occurs as a problem in isolation for adolescents. In addition, the adolescent may need help in other areas, such as physical disabilities, learning disabilities occurring as a result of molest, abuse, neglect, and sexual adjustment if he or she is to be able to focus on dealing with his or her substance abuse.

Some treatment facilities attempt to assess and deal with the wide variety of problems the adolescent may experience as a result of or in addition to substance abuse. However, this is not always the case and it is important for the referring physician to point out all of those areas in which significant problems are evident and to encourage seeking help in each of them.

Some referrals may be more acceptable to families than others. The diagnosis of adolescent or other drug abuse or dependency has become increasingly common in recent years. Many parents view this diagnosis as less stigmatizing than one of mental illness or chronic delinquency and therefore may be more willing to accept referral to a substance abuse treatment facility more readily than to family therapy, for example. It is important for the physician to use his or her expert authority and persuasive ability to encourage families to obtain help in all areas of need.

Range of Services Available

There is a wide variety of programs in existence to deal with alcohol and other drug-related problems in adolescence. These range from programs intended for intervention into early and emerging problems to those designed for dependent users.

Early intervention programs usually include a detailed assessment of the adolescents substance use and related problems. They may also include referral to services appropriate to problems that may be contributing to substance use. For example, if failure in school or family disruption appear to be related to the alcohol or other drug use, the adolescent may be referred to special school programs or to family therapy.

Early intervention programs may be associated with the schools, community mental health clinics, employee assistance programs (usually at the parent's place of work), juvenile courts, or they may be an outreach component of a treatment program.

If assessment indicates that the adolescent's alcohol or other drug-related problems are very severe or if the patient is dependent, entry into a treatment program may be called for. There are two general treatment modalities that are most suitable for adolescents: outpatient programs and residential programs. A third general type of treatment using such agonist drugs as methadone is generally not considered appropriate for adolescent patients, although antagonists, such as naltrexone or anabuse, are sometimes used as an adjunct to other forms of treatment. Within these modalities there is considerable variation in the type of setting and the degree of medical supervision.

The selection of a treatment setting should be made on the basis of an assessment of the patient's drug use patterns, level of dependency, and family and social situation. Cook and Petersen[19] suggested guidelines for individualizing the adolescent's treatment plan:

■ CRITERIA FOR SELECTING A TREATMENT SETTING

Criteria for Acute Hospital Care:

- Failure to progress in less intensive care settings.
- High-risk withdrawal (e.g., seizures, delirium tremens).
- High tolerance to one or more substances.

- Drug-related acute exacerbation of medical and/or psychiatric problems (e.g., cardiomyopathy, depression).
- Concomitant medical and/or psychiatric problems that could complicate treatment (e.g., diabetes, thought or character disorders).
- Severely impaired social, family or educational functioning.

Criteria for Partial Hospital Care:

- Does not require medically supervised withdrawal.
- Does not present with complicating medical and/or psychiatric problems.
- Able to function autonomously in non-residential setting; has intact social system (family, friends).
- Not in need of intensive psychiatric care.
- Free of psychoactive drugs other than prescribed medications.
- Requires daily rather than weekly support sessions.

Criteria for Non-Hospital Residential Care:

- Failure to progress in less intensive care settings.
- Withdrawal can be managed without close medical supervision.
- Has medical and/or psychiatric problems that are stable, but require monitoring.
- Has impaired social, family, or educational functioning that required separation from environment.
- Has sufficient interpersonal skills to function in milieu environment.

Criteria for Outpatient Care:

- Capable of functioning autonomously in present social environment.
- Has no acute medical and/or psychiatric problems.
- Has sufficient capacity to function in individual, group, and/or family therapy sessions.
- Withdrawal does not require medical supervision.

- Willing to work toward goal of abstinence from non-medical drug use.

■ OUTPATIENT PROGRAMS

Outpatient programs take a variety of forms ranging from unstructured drop-in centers to highly structured psychotherapy or family therapy. They also include activity programs, such as wilderness challenge experiences. Day treatment programs also fall into this category. These programs usually provide more intensive treatment and may fill 8 or more hours a day with therapeutic and educational activities. Day treatment programs are in many ways quite similar to residential treatment except that the patient returns home at night. In general, outpatient programs are less costly than residential programs.

■ HOSPITAL-BASED RESIDENTIAL TREATMENT

Residential treatment programs may include many of the same components as outpatient programs but in a more closely supervised and highly structured environment. The most common residential treatment programs are hospital based and typically last 4 weeks. They include group and individual counseling and are often based on the principles of Alcoholics Anonymous and Narcotics Anonymous.

Therapeutic Community

The second most common residential treatment model is the therapeutic community. This approach is based on the assumption that the drug-dependent person has never learned to function appropriately as an adolescent. Therefore, through the use of a highly structured, staged series of tasks and rewards, and through constant feedback from peers and counselors, the patient is socialized. The programs usually take place in a non-medical setting.

Often, privileges such as wearing one's own clothes, trips outside the facility, home visits, etc., are earned progressively. The group process tends to be confrontive in nature and is contraindicated in substance abusing clients who have severe psychiatric problems. Therapeutic communities may keep patients for as long as 2 years. For some individuals, particularly young adults, the therapeutic community may become a way of life, with ex-patients serving as staff members once the course of treatment is completed.

■ COMPARISON OF HOSPITAL AND THERAPEUTIC COMMUNITY MODELS

These two approaches tend to differ in the nature of training of program staff. The hospital-based programs include many staff with professional training and advanced degrees. Therapeutic communities, by contrast, depend to a large extent on paraprofessionals and staff who are themselves recovering addicts and who are assumed to have personal insight into the addiction process.

For adolescents, the exact nature of treatment to bring about the cessation of alcohol or other drug use may be less important than the additional services provided to prevent relapse and to deal with the other problems that drug abusing adolescents have. Adolescent patients differ from adults in a number of ways that must be dealt with in treatment. Adolescents have a higher incidence of family disorganization, are more likely to have emotional problems, sometimes including suicide attempts. They are also more likely to have remedial educational needs. In addition, normal developmental issues such as those related to sexuality and choice of vocation must be dealt with in this age group.

The most effective programs will incorporate aftercare planning into the program itself and will include an aggressive aftercare component once the program has been completed. Some of the features that seem most important include:

- An educational component which includes remedial education and the use of techniques to maximize achievement.

- Involvement of parents or significant others in the program so that they can provide support both during and after the program.
- Active leisure in areas of interest to the patient which can be sustained following program completion.
- Special services to address the individual needs of the patient, including mental health services, vocational counseling, sex education, and counseling, etc.
- Program components dealing with drug cravings, identification of high-risk situations, and handling relapse.

Managing Long-Term Care

Most treatment programs for adolescents have been shown to reduce alcohol and other drug use during treatment. However, programs have had less success in maintaining these reductions over the long run. Thus, any practitioner involved with the long-term care of alcohol and other drug-dependent adolescents must deal with the issue of relapse. Frequently, the process of reintegrating treated patients into home, school, and community and of providing the needed supports to prevent relapse is not given sufficient attention. Most relapses occur within the first 3 months following treatment. However, it has been suggested that adequate relapse prevention must include a commitment of 12–24 months of follow-up.[20]

Levels of Severity of Alcohol and Drug Problems

Level 1: *Experiencing social, legal, financial, or physical conse-quences of alcohol or drug abuse* (little or no dependence or serious medical or psychological complications)
Treatment Recommendations:
a. Trial of abstinence without medicated detoxification

b. Referral to counseling and AA/NA

c. Recheck in one week.

Level 2:   *Experiencing consequences of alcohol and drug abuse,*
           with signs of dependence and medical or psychological
           complications (intact social setting with supportive
           family, friends and co-workers)
           Treatment Recommendations:
           a. Outpatient detoxification, with daily monitoring and
              medication
           b. Referral to counseling and AA/NA
           c. Recheck and reevaluate in one week.

Level 3:   *Experiencing the same problems as Level 2, but without*
           24-hour social support (has no history of relapse)
           Treatment Recommendations:
           a. Inpatient detoxification and outpatient rehabilitation
           b. Referral to counseling and AA/NA
           c. Recheck and reevaluate in one week.

Level 4:   *Experiencing the same problems as Level 3; also has a*
           history of rapid release when treated in an out-patient
           program (has no history of relapse when treated in a
           short-term inpatient program)
           Treatment Recommendations:
           a. Inpatient detoxification and short-term inpatient reha-
              bilitation, with outpatient follow-up
           b. Referral to counseling and AA/NA
           c. Recheck in three weeks or upon discharge.

Level 5:   *Experiencing the same problems as Level 3; also has a*
           history of rapid relapse after short-term inpatient treat-
           ment
           Treatment Recommendations:
           a. Inpatient detoxification and long-term residential
              treatment
           b. Recheck in six months or upon discharge.

REFERENCES

1. Ehrlich P: Discussion of Adolescent Chemical Dependency Treatment. Unpublished manuscript, 1998.
2. Weston A: *The Wounded Healer: Power and Vulnerability.* Berkeley, CA: Saturday Seminar Series, 1989.
3. Miller A: *Drama of the Gifted Child.* New York: Basic Books, 1981.
4. Cermak T: *Diagnosing and Treating Codependence.* Minneapolis, MN: Johnson Institute, 1986.
5. Morrison MA, Smith DE, Wilford BB, Ehrlich P, Seymour RB: At war in the fields of play: current perspectives on the nature and treatment of adolescent chemical dependency, *Journal of Psychoactive Drugs,* 1993; 25(4): 321–330.
6. Wilford BB: *Kaiser Family Foundation Report on Capacity Building in Southern States.* Oakland, CA: Kaiser Family Foundation, 1994.
7. Seymour RB, Smith DE: *Drugfree: A Unique, Positive Approach to Staying Off Alcohol and Other Drugs.* New York: Facts on File Publications, 1987.
8. Seymour RB, Smith DE, Inaba DS, Landry M: *The New Drugs: Look-Alikes, Drugs of Deception and Designer Drugs.* Center City, MN: Hazelden, 1989.
9. Smith DE, Ehrlich P, Seymour RB: *Diagnosis and Treatment of the Adolescent Addict and Substance Abuser.* Unpublished Manuscript, 2000.
10. Klitzner M, Schwartz RH, Gruenewald P: Screening for risk factors for adolescent alcohol and drug use. *American Journal of Diseases of Children,* 1987; 141: 45–49.
11. Johnston LD, O'Malley PM, Bachman JG: *Illicit Drug Use, Smoking, and Drinking by America's High School Students, College Students and Young Adults, 1975-1987* (DHHS Pub. No. ADM 89-1602). Rockville, MD: National Institute on Drug Abuse, 1988.
12. Goodstadt MS: *Alcohol and Drug Education.* Health Education Monographs 1978; 6: 263–279.
13. Fuller PG, Cavanough RM: Basic assessment and screening for substance abuse in the pediatrician's office. *Pediatric Clinics of North America,* 1994; 42(2): 295–315.
14. Cavanaugh RM, Pickett M, Rogers PD: Screening for substance abuse in children and adolescents, in: Graham AW, Schultz TK, Wilford BB (eds.), *Principles of Addiction Medicine,* 2nd ed. Chevy

Chase, MD: American Society of Addiction Medicine, 1998, p. 1129.

15. Schwartz RH, Wirtz PW: Potential substance abuse: detection among adolescent patients. *Clinical Pediatrics* 1990; 29:38–43.
16. Comerci GD: Office assessment and brief intervention with the adolescent suspected of substance abuse, in: Graham AW, Schultz TK, Wilford BB (eds.), *Principles of Addiction Medicine,* 2nd ed. Chevy Chase, MD: American Society of Addiction Medicine, 1998, p. 1145.
17. Winters KC; Henley G: Assessing adolescents who abuse chemicals: The Chemical Dependency Adolescent Assessment Project, in: ER Rahdert, J Grabowski (eds.), *Adolescent Drug Abuse: Analyses of Treatment Research* (Research Monograph 77). Rockville, MD: National Institute on Drug Abuse, 1988.
18. Schuckit MA: *Drug and Alcohol Abuse: A Clinical Guide to Diagnosis and Treatment,* 3rd Ed. New York, NY: Plenum Medical Books, 1990.
19. Cook PS, Petersen RC: Individualizing adolescent drug abuse treatment, in: AS Friedman, GM Beschner (eds.), *Treatment Services for Adolescent Substance Abusers.* Rockville, MD: National Institute on Drug Abuse, 1985.
20. MacDonald DI: Substance abuse. *Pediatric Review*, 1988; 10: 89–94.

12

Chapter Twelve

Nutrition Counseling and Other Concerns in Supporting Recovery

Moving from drug dependency to recovery involves more than simply not taking drugs. Improving physical condition through nutrition, exercise and relaxation also improves the recovering patient's attitude and general well being, decreasing the potential for relapse into active addiction. Generally, drug abuse and addiction are antithetical to good nutrition. As a rule, the addicts diet is way out of balance. Eating may be sporadic, with an emphasis on sugars, animal protein and highly processed fast foods. The patient may have no clear sense of what constitutes good nutrition, and the therapist can play a vital role in providing information and direction toward physical rehabilitation through proper diet.

Improving a Patient's Diet

The best way to start is by taking a good look at the patient's present diet. Have him or her make a list of what has been eaten in the course of a week and discuss ingredients and food preparation. Pay particular attention to the ingredients of any processed foods used by the patient. Note that these ingredients appear on the label by order of quantity, the highest quantity listed first. You and the patient may be amazed at the number of products in which the first or second ingredient is sugar, salt, or high fructose corn syrup, all conductive to hypertension, and how often hydrogenated or partially hydrogenated oils appear on the labels.

If patients do their own cooking, suggest that they try to use fewer processed and preserved foods and more natural ingredients. Fresh fruits and vegetables are becoming more available even in urban environments, and cooking with them may increase time in the kitchen but the results are worth it. There are increasing number of good cookbooks on the market that emphasize easy-to-make dishes with fresh ingredients.

Patients who eat in restaurants can be advised to watch for restaurants that emphasize grains, legumes (including beans, lentils, peas), vegetables, fruits, nuts, and seeds on their menus, and to avoid deep-fried foods and dishes that are heavy in meat and dairy products.

As ours has become more of an urban society in which most people buy their food in stores rather than growing it, foods have become increasingly processed and refined. In the interest of health, the recovering individual may have to seek out less refined options. Instead of white bread or refined "whole wheat" bread, substitute whole-grain bread, preferably stone ground to decrease their highly soluble lipoprotein content, made from wheat, rye, rice, corn, millet oats, buckwheat, and/or barley. Whole-grain pastas are also available. Substitute brown rice for white and olive oil or canola oil for butter, margarine and other oils in cooking and salad dressings. Eat salads!

One bonus is that natural foods taste better. They may not seem to at first, especially if one is used to a steady diet of pizazzed fast food that is overloaded with flavor additives. Processed foods often contain chemicals that affect one's tastebuds in the same way that drugs effect the brain, leaving them insensitive to natural flavors. Many drugs, such as nicotine, cocaine, caffeine and alcohol, also deaden our ability to smell and taste, and it may take a while to regain these senses.

Establishing the right diet with the right nutrition often depends on the patient's location and circumstances. Fresh and natural foods will be easier to find if they live on a full-service farm than if they live in a downtown hotel room, surrounded by golden arches and plastic cups. Mainly, it involves paying attention to what is available. Canned soups, for example, can be remarkably free from additives and preservatives, but there are exceptions. Urge patients to read all labels and question anything that seems unfamiliar. Urge them to seek out health food stores and restaurants and not to be afraid to ask questions about nutrition. The people who work in these places are often there because they are interested in good nutrition and are more than willing to help.[1]

Eating Disorders

Often the addicted individual is also a victim of eating disorders, and when these are present it is up to the therapist to work with these problems as well as the primary addiction. Eating disorders bear a close similarity to substance abuse and addiction. Using a 12-Step approach, Overeaters Anonymous has been successful in dealing with a number of problems and some clinical ecologists, such as Theron G. Randolph and Ralph W. Moss[2] suggest that food addiction and drug addiction may be closely related. Scientists studying anorexia nervosa and bulimia have seen close correlations between these puzzling diseases and addiction as well.

The relationships between nutrition, addiction, and behavior can manifest in a number of ways. Deficiencies in nutrients, for example, can cause problems and can result from both intake and utilization. An individual may have adequate intake of a needed vitamin or amino acid, but the substance is blocked from getting to the tissue that needs it by poor digestion, malabsorption, or biochemical defects in the system. Scientists are now learning that proper digestion of one nutrient often depends on the presence of certain others.

Appetite control mechanisms in the brain have an effect on our intake of both food and drugs. To an extent, the action of these mechanisms is dependent on one's nutritional status, or "What you eat and drink is determined by what you eat and drink."[3]

Nutrition, however, does not exist in a vacuum any more than any other factor in abuse and addiction. It has to be considered along with everything else. Also, poor nutrition may be a cause for many problems that can exacerbate abuse and addiction or interfere with recovery. These problems can include sexual inadequacy, social inadequacy, chronic pain, inability to cope with stress, lack of control over thoughts, feelings or actions, depression, anxiety, and poor self-esteem. These are symptoms that often involve unstable blood sugar, food allergy, nutrient deficiencies, or other aspects of nutritional imbalance.

The following are 12 treatment goals in which the therapist can interact with the patient toward physical recovery:

1. *Elimination of nutritional deficiencies*: Stress, history of poor diet, exposure to toxins, pollutants or allergens, chronic disease and recovery from disease, injury or surgery greatly increase the risk of deficiency and therefore increase the risk for sluggish functioning of the body's healing mechanisms. Deficiency is a relative matter, and large doses of certain nutrients are sometimes required to eliminate a deficiency.

2. *Treatment of hypoglycemia*: Nearly all alcoholics in early recovery experience functional hypoglycemia, i.e., they experience blood sugar instability or low blood sugar to some extent. Dietary treatment of this condition is critical for optimum recovery.

3. *Identification of food allergies, addictions or hypersensitivities*: Many foods trigger symptoms that lead to or intensify a desire to drink. For an alcoholic, these foods may be those from which his or her favorite beverage is made. Identification and elimination of such foods can be critical to easier sobriety and optimum recovery.

4. *Repair of damaged tissues and organs*: Certain tissues can either regenerate or repair themselves. The efficiency of this process depends upon optimum nutritional intake.

5. *Restoration of function of vital systems*: Stress, poor diet and chronic illness can affect vital systems in ways that are mani-

fested through symptoms and in ways that are not. Restoration of these systems, which include the brain, heart, liver, endocrine system and immune system, is critical to recovery and depend on optimum nutrition more than on any other single factor.

6. *Reduction of craving for alcohol, sugar, caffeine, and nicotine*: Cravings, to a large extent, result from lack of nutritional integrity and from dietary intake that is neither balanced nor centered. A positive approach to reducing your cravings is based upon building nutritional integrity through nutrient supplementation and through a balanced and centered diet.

7. *Restoration of appetite*: Ironically, your nutritional status is a determinant of your appetite, and appetite affects what you eat. The hypothalamus is generally understood to be the center of appetite control (it is also the center of emotional control, which is related to appetite). Brain function depends critically on nutritional status. In addition, imbalance in some nutrients can inhibit the senses of taste and smell. Thus, we can expect our appetite for nourishing food to increase as our nutritional status is improved.

8. *Restoration of initiative, confidence, and willingness to cooperate*: The awakening of cognitive function, feelings, positive self-image and positive interpersonal interactions will result in varying degrees from nutritional therapy. These changes often lead to increased initiative, confidence, and cooperation in the treatment process. No one, of course, can predict the extent of response to therapy, but good nutrition can accomplish a great deal.

9. *Increased ability to handle stress*: The strain on a person depends on the extent to which an event is perceived as stressful and on the extent to which the body's various systems—central nervous system, endocrine, etc.—are taxed by the resulting stress. Our nutritional integrity is a factor in the experience of stress as well as in our body's defensive and restorative functions. Dietary intake itself can be a major source of stress (sugar, caffeine, toxins, allergens), or it can provide protection against stress.

10. *Creation of less internal (digestive, metabolic) stress.* The intake of harmful foods and chemicals and the resulting digestive and metabolic chaos can be as intense a source of stress as any that you experience. Digestive and metabolic stress lead to a vicious cycle. The more of this stress you experience, the less value is gotten from the very food and supplements necessary to improve functioning of your digestive and metabolic systems. Nutritional therapy can turn this downward spiral into an upward, healing cycle.

11. *Minimization of withdrawal symptoms*: A certain stress is associated with withdrawal from any addictive substance. Withdrawal symptoms are the most obvious part of the difficulties associated with abstinence and management of cravings. There is a growing body of evidence demonstrating that withdrawal symptoms in particular, and the experience of pain in general, are lessened by improving nutritional status. Withdrawal can be even easier if you prepare for it by building your nutritional status prior to withdrawal.

12. *Treatment of diseases associated with substance abuse*: Because of the general deterioration of all of the body's systems, including the immune system, there are endless possibilities for the occurrence of physical, mental and emotional dysfunction as a result of substance abuse. The function of nutritional therapy, again is support of the body's own efforts to heal itself and restore balance.[3]

Treatment centers, such as the Haight Ashbury Free Clinics in San Francisco, are beginning to incorporate nutritional counseling into their treatment protocols. In the *Principles of Addiction Medicine,* Lawrence Feinman and Charles S. Lieber[4] discuss the relation of alcoholism and nutrition, pointing out that for heavy drinkers, ethanol may provide more than half the daily energy needs.

Conversely, James Smith[5] points out that chronic alcohol and other drug use can lead to decreased intake and absorption of vitamins, amino acids, and fats through alcohol damage to the intestine and/or pancreas.

Some Final Thoughts About Recovery ....

In many ways, the concerned health professional provides the link between active addiction and active recovery. The ability to perform this service adequately and skillfully depends on knowledge and understanding of the key factors involved and a professional willingness to go the distance in helping a patient into his or her own remission. In the end, there is only so much that the physician/therapist can do. The real work of recovery is up to the recovering individual. That does not mean, however, that the physician does not play an important and ongoing role in solidifying and enhancing the patient's recovery.

As you have seen in this book, there are many issues involved in treatment and recovery both on the short and the long term. In treatment, it is important to be thorough. Dual diagnosis, or as some therapists are now calling it full spectrum mental disorders including substance abuse and addiction, is a factor in many cases. Issues of anxiety and depression can sabotage both treatment and recovery. Physical disease and drug abuse sequelae can be hiding within the acute diagnosis. Family and individual history can provide important clues to treatment needs. Be thorough.

As John Chappel[6] pointed out in Chapter 7, it is important for the therapist to be familiar with the nature of recovery and be ready to help the patient find his or her niche or niches within the web of recovery fellowships. Addiction is a physical, mental and spiritual disease and needs to be treated as such. Please become familiar with the A.A., N.A., CA, SOS, Rational Recovery, etc., meetings in your vicinity and even attend a few. Much of the progress that has been made in the field has been through the recognition of the value of self-help, and attending a few meetings can be a revelation for the practitioner.

Finally, in this book the authors have addressed you via a number of titles: physician, therapist, practitioner, etc. For the purpose of this text, all of these are interchangeable. The nature of this book is to provide information on the treatment of drug abuse and addiction to the health professional of whatever discipline who has not had specialist training in addiction medicine. For that matter, specialists may even find materials of value in these pages. Much, much more detailed information on addiction treatment is available from the American Society of Addiction Medicine and their fine, definitive text *Principles of Addiction Medicine, Second Edition.*

The authors wish you well.

REFERENCES

1. Seymour RB, Smith DE: *Drugfree: A Unique, Positive Approach to Staying Off Alcohol and Other Drugs.* New York: Facts on File Publications/Sarah Lazin Books, 1987.
2. Randolph TG, Moss RW. *An Alternative Approach to Allergies: The New Field of Clinical Ecology Unravels the Environmental Causes of Mental and Physical Ills.* New York: Harper and Row Publishers, Inc., 1980.
3. Land DR: *Eat Right!* Center City, MN: Hazelden, 1985.
4. Feinman L, Lieber CS. Nutrition, in: Graham AW, Schultz TK, Wilford BB (eds.), *Principles of Addiction Medicine,* 2nd ed. Chevy Chase, MD: American Society of Addiction Medicine, 1998, p. 741.
5. Smith JW: Special problems of the elderly, in: Graham AW, Schultz TK, Wilford BB (eds.), *Principles of Addiction Medicine,* 2nd ed. Chevy Chase, MD: American Society of Addiction Medicine, 1998, p. 833.
6. Chappel JN: Spiritual components of the recovery process, in: Graham AW, Schultz TK, Wilford BB (eds.), *Principles of Addiction Medicine,* 2nd ed. Chevy Chase, MD: American Society of Addiction Medicine, 1998, p. 725.

I

Appendix I

American Society of Addiction Medicine Patient Placement Criteria

ADULT ADMISSION CRITERIA: CROSSWALK OF LEVELS 0.5 THROUGH IV

			Levels of Service		
Criteria Dimensions	Level 0.5 Early Intervention	Opioid Maintenance Therapy	Level I Outpatient Services	Level II.1 Intensive Outpatient	Level II.5 Partial Hospitalization
DIMENSION 1: Alcohol Intoxication and/or Withdrawal Potential	No withdrawal risk	Patient is physiologically dependent on opiates and requires OMT to prevent withdrawal	I-D, Ambulatory detoxification without extended on-site monitoring Minimal risk of severe withdrawal	Minimal risk of severe withdrawal	II-D, Ambulatory detoxification with extended on-site monitoring Moderate risk of severe withdrawal
DIMENSION 2: Biomedical Conditions and Complications	None or very stable	None or manageable with outpatient medical monitoring	None or very stable	None or not a distraction from treatment and manageable in Level II.1	None or not sufficient to distract from treatment and manageable in Level II.5
DIMENSION 3: Emotional, Behavioral, or Cognitive Conditions and Complications	None or very stable	None or manageable in outpatient structured environment	None or very stable	Mild severity, with potential to distract from recovery; needs monitoring	Mild to moderate severity, with potential to distract from recovery; needs stabilization

DIMENSION 4: Readiness to Change	Willing to understand how current use may affect personal goals	Resistance high enough to require structured therapy to promote treatment progress but will not render outpatient treatment ineffective	Willing to cooperate but needs motivating and monitoring strategies	Resistance high enough to require structured program but not so high as to render outpatient treatment ineffective	Resistance high enough to require structured program but not so high as to render outpatient treatment ineffective
DIMENSION 5: Relapse, Continued Use, or Continued Problem Potential	Needs understanding of, or skills to change, current use patterns	High risk of relapse or continued use without OMT and structured therapy to promote treatment progress	Able to maintain abstinence or control use and pursue recovery goals with minimal support	Intensification of addiction symptoms, despite active participation in Level I, and high likelihood of relapse or continued use without close monitoring and support	Intensification of addiction symptoms, despite active participation in Level I or II.1; high likelihood of relapse or continued use without monitoring and support
DIMENSION 6: Recovery Environment	Social support system or significant others increase risk for personal conflict about alcohol/drug use	Supportive recovery environment and/or patient has skills to cope with outpatient treatment	Supportive recovery environment and/or patient has skills to cope	Environment unsupportive, but with structure and support the patient can cope	Environment is not supportive but, with structure and support and relief from the home environment, the patient can cope

ADULT ADMISSION CRITERIA: CROSSWALK OF LEVELS 0.5 THROUGH IV (continued)

Criteria Dimensions	Level III.1 Clinically Managed Low-Intensity Residential Services	Level III.3 Clinically Managed Medium-Intensity Residential Services	Level III.5 Clinically Managed High-Intensity Residential Services	Level III.7 Medically Monitored Intensive Inpatient Services	Level IV Medically Managed Intensive Inpatient Services
			Levels of Service		
DIMENSION 1: Alcohol Intoxication and/or Withdrawal Potential	No withdrawal risk	Level III.2-D, Clinically Managed Residential Detoxification Services No severe withdrawal risk, but moderate withdrawal manageable in III.2-D	Minimal risk of severe withdrawal for Level III.3 and III.5. If withdrawal is present, meets Level III.2-D criteria	III.7-D, Medically Monitored Inpatient Detoxification Services Severe withdrawal, but manageable in Level III.7-D	IV-D, Medically Managed Inpatient Detoxification Services Severe withdrawal risk
DIMENSION 2: Biomedical Conditions and Complications	None or stable	None or stable	None or stable; receiving concurrent medical monitoring	Patient requires medical monitoring but not intensive treatment	Patient requires 24-hour medical and nursing care
DIMENSION 3: Emotional, Behavioral, or Cognitive Conditions and Complications	None or minimal; not distracting to recovery	Mild to moderate severity; needs structure to allow focus on recovery	Repeated inability to control impulses; personality disorder requires high structure to shape behavior	Moderate severity; patient needs a 24-hour structured setting	Severe problems require 24-hour psychiatric care with concomitant addiction treatment

DIMENSION 4: Readiness to Change	Open to recovery, but needs structured environment to maintain therapeutic gains	Little awareness; patient needs interventions available only in Level III.3 to engage and keep in treatment	Market difficulty with or opposition to treatment, with dangerous consequences if not engaged in treatment	Resistance high and impulse control poor, despite negative consequences; patient needs motivating strategies available only in 24-hour structured setting	Problems in this dimension do not qualify the patient for Level IV services
DIMENSION 5: Relapse, Continued Use, or Continued Problem Potential	Understands relapse but needs structure to maintain therapeutic gains	Little awareness; patient needs interventions available only in Level III.3 to prevent continued use	No recognition of skills needed to prevent continued use, with dangerous consequences	Unable to control use, with dangerous consequences, despite active participation in less intensive care	Problems in this dimension do not qualify the patient for Level IV services
DIMENSION 6: Recovery Environment	Environment is dangerous, but recovery achievable if Level III.1 structure is available	Environment is dangerous; patient needs 24-hour structure to learn to cope	Environment dangerous; patient lacks skills to cope outside of a highly structured 24-hour setting	Environment dangerous for recovery; patient lacks skills to cope outside of highly structured 24-hour setting	Problems in this dimension do not qualify the patient for Level IV services

Note: This overview of the Adult Admission Criteria is an approximate summary to illustrate the principal concepts and structure of the criteria.

Crosswalk excerpted from the *ASAM Patient Placement Criteria for the Treatment of Substance-Related Disorders*, Second Edition-Revised (ASAM PPC-2R). Copyright 2001, American Society of Addiction Medicine, Chevy Chase, MD.

II

Resources for Consultation and Referral

When a patient presents with what may be substance abuse or addiction, there are many questions and concerns. Can I treat this individual? That is a very good question. Doctors responding to a series of studies conducted by Dr. John Chappel and reported in *Drugfree*[1] indicated that they would go out of their way not to treat anyone they suspected of abuse or addiction. Further, many current laws governing the practice of medicine reinforce this predilection by subjecting physicians who do treat abusers and addicts to intense scrutiny by enforcement agencies and peer review boards that often share the general lack of knowledge about abuse and addiction.

Acting out of fear, ignorance or prejudice, physicians will often miss a primary diagnosis involving alcohol or other drugs. They may miss the primary cause of stress in the home or a history of accidents and minor illnesses. At times they will prescribe the very drugs that can lead to an exacerbation of the problem. Misprescription often results from a doctor losing touch or not keeping up with developments in pharmacology.

As a consequence, treatment has primarily been in the hands of licensed specialty agencies such as methadone maintenance clinics, hospital drug wards, therapeutic communities, etc. With increasing treatment waiting lists around the country, the treatment of abuse and addiction is having to move into mainstream medicine, and legislation is pointing toward a more open use of nonspecialists employing such medications as methadone, buprenorphine and naltrexone in protocols that can be maintained in an office setting. However, it will be important for participating physicians to become knowledgeable and proficient in order to provide such treatment.

Training Opportunities

In conjunction with many colleagues, your authors have developed and presented continuing medical education courses in prescribing practices that are aimed at the nonspecialist. In many states, physicians are required to take a certain number of educational units per year as part of their license requirements. These courses include updates on the nature of all psychoactive drugs, guides to diagnosis, alternatives to and strategies for prescribing psychoactive medications, role play on dealing with prescription scams, and attitudinal work.

Today, continuing education programs have proliferated to the point where the potential attendee/client needs to literally separate the wheat from the chaff. In selecting continuing education venues, it is important to find those with presenters who have validity and standing in the field and who are presenting on specific topics that will aid your understanding and ability to provide treatment. Watch for courses that are sponsored by bona fide state and national medical education entities. In California, for example, courses that provide Category 1 CME and display the seal of the California Medical Association and contain the wording, "This is an activity offered by _____ a California Medical Association accredited provider. Physicians may report up to _ hours of Category 1 credits toward the California Medical Association's Certificate in Continuing Medical Education and the American Medical Association's Physician's Recognition Award," have the highest quality of content and value to the physician. Other national and state bodies provide credit for nurses, MFT/LCSWs, counselors, psychologists, etc. Most credit is awarded by state levels but recognized nationally and therefore by other states.

In many areas, colleges and universities have substance abuse programs that may range from one-course extended education programs to full curriculums covering several years of in-classroom work and practicum.

Internet Information

There is much information to be found on the internet, but here too the proliferation has created a tower of misinformation as well. Government sources are probably the best and most reliable and most drug-related agencies have extensive web sites. These include sites for the Substance Abuse and Mental Health Services Administration (SAMHSA), the National Institute on Drug Abuse (NIDA), the National Institute on Alcoholism and Alcohol Abuse (NIAAA), the Center for Substance Abuse Treatment (CSAT), and the Center for Substance Abuse Prevention (CSAP). All of these have newsletters and publish manuals and other materials listed and with access information on their sites.

AlcoholMD.com

A new web page that your authors recommend highly, in part because we are its editors, is AlcoholMD.com. The page is set up in three parts: professional information, information for the general public, and information for children. The professional segment contains much useful information on addiction and treatment as well as a regularly updated International Addictions Infoline and a "Yellow Pages" of information on treatment sites and the services that they offer. AlcoholMD.com is sponsored by DrugAbuse Sciences, Inc., a producer of medications for the treatment of alcoholism and other drug addiction dedicated to the "enhancement" not the replacement of treatment.

AMERICAN SOCIETY OF ADDICTION MEDICINE

Probably the best source of professional information on addiction and treatment is the American Society of Addiction Medicine, Inc., 4601 North Park Avenue, Suite 101, Chevy Chase, MD 20815. Telephone 301 656 3620, Fax 301 656 3815, e-mail: email@asam.org. ASAM produces a regular newsletter.

OTHER SOURCES FOR CONSULTATION AND REFERRAL

Each state has a state agency that provides support and coordination for research, prevention, and treatment providers within the state. In California, that is the State of California Department of Health Alcohol and Drug Programs (ADP), located at 1700 "K" Street, Sacramento, CA 95814. Generally, there is an agency for each subdivision within each state, whether it be a county, ward, or whatever, that coordinates services within its precincts. The county agencies are probably the best first line of information of public treatment entities but may be less helpful on private non-supported programs. For physicians, your county or state medical society is a good source of information. At the national level, CSAT now has a directory of over 6,000 treatment sources on its web page that is updated annually.

REFERENCES

1. Seymour RB, Smith DE: *Drugfree: A Unique, Positive Approach to Staying Off Alcohol and Other Drugs.* New York: Facts on File Publications, 1987.

Index

ISBN 0-07-134713-5

90000

SMITH/SUBSTANCE ABUSE